Managing Bipolar Disorder

✓ Treatments *That Work*™

Managing Bipolar Disorder

A COGNITIVE-BEHAVIORAL APPROACH

Therapist Guide

Michael W. Otto • Noreen A. Reilly-Harrington
Jane N. Kogan • Aude Henin • Robert O. Knauz
Gary S. Sachs

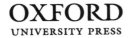

OXFORD
UNIVERSITY PRESS

2009

OXFORD
UNIVERSITY PRESS

Oxford University Press, Inc., publishes works that further
Oxford University's objective of excellence
in research, scholarship, and education.

Oxford   New York
Auckland   Cape Town   Dar es Salaam   Hong Kong   Karachi
Kuala Lumpur   Madrid   Melbourne   Mexico City   Nairobi
New Delhi   Shanghai   Taipei   Toronto

With offices in
Argentina   Austria   Brazil   Chile   Czech Republic   France   Greece
Guatemala   Hungary   Italy   Japan   Poland   Portugal   Singapore
South Korea   Switzerland   Thailand   Turkey   Ukraine   Vietnam

Copyright © 2009 by Oxford University Press, Inc.

Published by Oxford University Press, Inc.
198 Madison Avenue, New York, New York 10016

www.oup.com

Oxford is a registered trademark of Oxford University Press

Library of Congress Cataloging-in-Publication Date

CIP data on file

ISBN 978-0-19-531334-5

9 8 7 6 5 4 3 2 1

Printed in the United States of America

About Treatments *ThatWork*™

Stunning developments in healthcare have taken place over the last several years, but many of our widely accepted interventions and strategies in mental health and behavioral medicine have been brought into question by research evidence as not only lacking benefit, but perhaps, inducing harm. Other strategies have been proven effective using the best current standards of evidence, resulting in broad-based recommendations to make these practices more available to the public. Several recent developments are behind this revolution. First, we have arrived at a much deeper understanding of pathology, both psychological and physical, which has led to the development of new, more precisely targeted interventions. Second, our research methodologies have improved substantially, such that we have reduced threats to internal and external validity, making the outcomes more directly applicable to clinical situations. Third, governments around the world and health care systems and policymakers have decided that the quality of care should improve, that it should be evidence based, and that it is in the public's interest to ensure that this happens (Barlow, 2004; Institute of Medicine, 2001).

Of course, the major stumbling block for clinicians everywhere is the accessibility of newly developed evidence-based psychological interventions. Workshops and books can go only so far in acquainting responsible and conscientious practitioners with the latest behavioral healthcare practices and their applicability to individual patients. This new series, Treatments *ThatWork*™, is devoted to communicating these exciting new interventions to clinicians on the frontlines of practice.

The manuals and workbooks in this series contain step-by-step detailed procedures for assessing and treating specific problems and diagnoses. But this series also goes beyond the books and manuals by providing ancillary materials that will approximate the supervisory process in assisting practitioners in the implementation of these procedures in their practice.

In our emerging healthcare system, the growing consensus is that evidence-based practice offers the most responsible course of action for the mental health professional. All behavioral healthcare clinicians deeply desire to provide the best possible care for their patients. In this series, our aim is to close the dissemination and information gap and make that possible.

This therapist guide addresses the management of bipolar disorder. Divided into four phases, this 30-session program is designed to be used in conjunction with pharmacotherapy and focuses on helping the patient alleviate depressive episodes, form a support system of family and friends, focus on the most relevant problems outside of the disorder, and improve well-being. The program is based on the principles of CBT and includes such skills as cognitive restructuring, problem solving, mood charting, and activity scheduling. A major goal of the program is the creation of a Treatment Contract that informs the patient's treatment team and support network how to recognize possible periods of illness and the strategies they should use in order to help the patient during these times.

Complete with step-by-step instructions for running sessions, as well as lists of materials needed, session outlines, and copies of forms necessary for treatment, this therapist guide provides you with all the information you need to help your bipolar patients successfully manage the disorder.

David H. Barlow, Editor-in-Chief,
Treatments *ThatWork*™
Boston, MA

References

Barlow, D. H. (2004). Psychological treatments. *American Psychologist, 59,* 869–878.

Institute of Medicine. (2001). *Crossing the quality chasm: A new health system for the 21st century.* Washington, DC: National Academy Press.

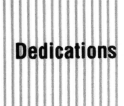

Dedications

MWO: For my brother Ken and his family, for your love

NAR-H: For my husband, my parents, and my three precious sons, with all my love

JNK: For my husband Evan, for the love and levity in every day

AH: For the ones who guide and inspire me: my parents, my husband, and my children

ROK: For my son Lucas, who completed the circle of our family

GSS: To James, Leslie, and Gregory, for their endless inspiration and generous patience

Acknowledgements

This book was designed for clinicians treating individuals with bipolar disorder. It provides a wealth of information and step-by-step clinical strategies for the management of bipolar disorder. These strategies were shaped by our collaborations with a number of teams of clinicians and clinical researchers as well as by the patients with whom we have worked. For their early work, we would like to thank and acknowledge the input from Dina Hirshfeld-Becker and Robert Gould, who initiated a program of group CBT for bipolar disorder at Massachusetts General Hospital. We would also like to thank our collaborators in the Systematic Treatment Enhancement Program for Bipolar Disorder (STEP-BD). Our perspectives on treatment were further influenced by the treatment methods and/or independent studies led by Judith Beck, Aaron T. Beck, Ellen Frank, Dominic Lam, Robert Leahy, David Miklowitz, Cory Newman, Jan Scott, and Ari Zaretsky. Likewise, we learned the value of attending to the promotion of well-being from research by Giovanni Fava. We thank all of these individuals for their valuable input and expanding what is known about the nature and treatment of bipolar disorder.

Contents

Chapter 1   *Introductory Information for Therapists*

Background Information and Purpose of This Program

This treatment manual is designed for use by therapists in the management of bipolar disorder. In structuring this manual, we utilized information from clinical trials and our clinical experience to provide instruction in a flexibly applied cognitive-behavioral approach to treating bipolar disorder across phases of the illness, with attention to the treatment of core symptoms of depression as well as the management of factors shown to be important in predicting relapse.

Therapists providing this treatment will recognize interventions as an expansion of cognitive-behavioral strategies (namely informational interventions, cognitive restructuring, and behavioral activation) for *unipolar* depression, combined with interventions specific to the issues and difficulties confronting individuals with bipolar disorder. The manual is designed for use with patients in the depressive phase of the disorder, as well as those needing relapse-prevention efforts once initial mood stabilization is achieved. Relapse-prevention efforts involve psychoeducation on the nature of bipolar disorder, including risk and resilience factors and the importance of medication adherence; activity and lifestyle regulation combined with stress management; training in problem solving; training in interpersonal skills; and planning for the early identification and intervention with prodromal symptoms of both depression and (hypo)mania. This treatment is designed to accompany ongoing pharmacotherapy for bipolar disorder and is expected to treat bipolar depression, as well as aid mood stabilization over and above the effects of pharmacotherapy and enhanced medication adherence.

Bipolar disorder and related conditions are estimated to affect between 1% and 5% of the population: over 10 million individuals in the United States (Akiskal, 2007; Kessler et al., 1994; McIntryre & Konarski, 2004). Age of onset of the disorder is typically in the mid-teens, with evidence for a worse course and greater comorbidity for individuals with a particularly early onset (Perlis et al., 2004). Bipolar disorder appears to strike women and men at approximately equal rates (Kessler et al., 1994), although the rapid cycling (four or more mood episodes a year) subtype of the disorder appears to be more common in women (Schneck et al., 2004).

The most common clinical course of bipolar disorder is characterized by repeated mood episodes that are compounded by the frequent occurrence of residual symptoms and impaired role functioning even during periods of relative recovery (Keck et al., 1998). Approximately three-quarters of patients can be expected to relapse at different year intervals, with most of these relapses occurring in the first year.

A number of factors are associated with an increased frequency and chronicity of mood episodes. Stressful family environments (as defined by high levels of expressed emotion) as well as stressful life events have been linked with both delayed recovery and elevated relapse rates (Ellicott, Hammen, Gitlin, Brown, & Jamison, 1990; Johnson & Miller, 1997; Kim, Miklowitz, Biuckians, & Mullen, 2007; Miklowitz, Goldstein, Nuechterlein, Snyder, & Mintz, 1988). Moreover, anxiety and substance use comorbidity is marked in bipolar disorder and is also associated with a poorer course. For example, anxiety comorbidity has been linked with a decreased likelihood of recovery from a mood episode, poorer role functioning and quality of life, less time euthymic, a greater likelihood of suicide attempts, and poorer response to at least one class of medications (Henry, Van den Bulke, Bellivier, Etan, Rouillon, & Leboyer, 2003; Otto et al., 2006; Simon et al., 2004). Studies have also documented poorer recovery, poorer medication compliance, and more hospitalizations among bipolar patients with comorbid substance use disorders (Goldberg, Garno, Leon, Kocsis, & Portera, 1999; Keck et al., 1996; Keller et al., 1986; Weiss et al., 2005). Elevated rates of attention deficit disorder and eating disorders have also been reported for samples of patients with bipolar disorder (McElroy et al., 2000; Nierenberg et al., 2005).

Suicide is also a particular concern for individuals with bipolar disorder. For example, as evaluated in a 20-year longitudinal study of nearly 7,000 psychiatric outpatients in Pennsylvania, Brown, Beck, Steer, and Grisham (2000) found that patients with bipolar disorder had the strongest risk for completed suicide. As compared to the average psychiatric patients in the sample, bipolar patients were found to have a nearly fourfold increase in suicide risk. The next highest risk was found for major depression, which accounted for a threefold increase in risk. Within samples of bipolar patients, duration of depression, amount of psychosocial stressors, and anxiety comorbidity (particularly anxious rumination) have been found to predict suicidal behavior, but a past history of suicide attempts appears to be a particularly reliable and powerful predictor of future attempts (Leverich et al., 2003; Marangell et al., 2006; Simon et al., 2007). Attention to all of these variables is warranted as part of ongoing clinical vigilance.

Diagnostic Criteria and Differential Diagnosis for Bipolar Disorder

Bipolar disorder is most commonly characterized by repeated episodes of major depression, and at least one manic or hypomanic episode. Bipolar subtype (I versus II) is defined by a history of mania versus hypomania. Bipolar I disorder is defined by at least one episode of mania, whereas the bipolar II subtype refers to individuals who have had at least one hypomanic, but not full manic, episode and one or more depressive episodes.

A full manic episode is defined by a period of 1 week (unless interrupted by treatment or other factors) of feeling euphoric, irritable, or high, along with three or more of the following symptoms: racing thoughts, distractibility, exaggerated feelings of importance, little need for sleep, pressured speech, and reckless behavior (American Psychiatric Association, 2000). Hypomanic episodes are similar to manic episodes, except that they are less severe and impairing. The characteristics of depressive episodes are identical to those that define major depression. Depression requires at least five symptoms, present for a minimum of 2 weeks, including at least one of the core symptoms of (1) depressed mood and (2) loss of interest in activity. A handy mnemonic for the symptoms of depression other than a depressed mood is SIG E CAPS, representing **S**leep disruptions, diminished **I**nterest or pleasure, **G**uilt, low **E**nergy, **C**oncentration difficulties, **A**ppetite (or weight) changes, **P**sychomotor retardation or agitation, and **S**uicidal behavior (personal communication, Carey Gross).

The most common course of bipolar disorder is repeated episodes of depression and mania or hypomania. Although there is wide individual variation in the pattern of episodes, depressive symptoms are generally much more common than manic or hypomanic symptoms (Judd et al., 2003a, b) and represent an especially impairing and chronic phase of the disorder. Nonetheless, because of engagement in reckless behavior with serious social and role consequences (e.g., reckless driving, sexual affairs, financial blunders, intoxication, and aggressive behavior), full manic episodes can have dramatic and long-term effects on functioning.

In individuals with a history of depression, the differential diagnosis of unipolar major depression versus bipolar disorder revolves around the identification of manic or hypomanic episodes. In addition, any apparent episodes of (hypo)mania need to be differentiated from other co-occurring conditions such as substance use disorders and cluster B personality disorders. For example, substance use disorders may lead to episodes of poor judgment and risky behaviors (e.g., reckless driving or unprotected sexual encounters), as well as loud or boisterous speech and aggressive or irritable behaviors. Likewise, mood lability, interpersonal sensitivity, and risky behaviors may be part of borderline or histrionic patterns rather than the more-discrete episodes of mood episode–dependent behavior occurring with hypomania or mania. Finally, differential diagnosis may be made more complex by the presence of any number of these conditions at once: for example, bipolar disorder and substance use disorder. Finally, the presence of psychosis as part of manic or depressive episodes presents additional diagnostic challenges, requiring the clinician to differentiate bipolar episodes with psychotic features from schizoaffective disorder or schizophrenia. Some of these issues are clarified only after the mood-state dependency of symptoms is clarified after periods of acute recovery.

A full clinical assessment of bipolar disorder needs to include assessment of each pole of the disorder (manic and depressive symptoms), the history of the frequency and duration of episodes, potential biological provocations of these episodes (e.g., drug use), family history of episodes, psychosocial stressors, support networks, sleep and activity patterns, and role functioning. Attention to the frequency and role of hostility and anger in relation to symptoms is also important, especially with respect to relationship stresses.

Family involvement in initial or follow-up assessments is frequently helpful because patients may minimize manic or hypomanic episodes ("Sure I was hyped up and irritable, but I was also making some important financial decisions and working really hard"). Records from previous health care providers or previous hospitalizations may aid in the characterization of the severity of mood episodes when they were occurring, as compared to the memory bias that may be present when these episodes are recalled months or years later. Finally, in relation to the review of past records, it is important to remember that bipolar disorder may emerge from a history of apparent recurrent *unipolar* depression. For example, Goldberg, Harrow, and Whiteside (2001) documented the later emergence of bipolar disorder in a proportion of individuals who were hospitalized for severe unipolar depression in adolescence.

Careful diagnostic assessment can be aided by the use of a semistructured interview such as the Structured Clinical Interview for DSM-IV Axis I diagnosis (SCID-I/P; First, Spitzer, Gibbon, & Williams, 2002). By specifying the minimum questions to be asked, the SCID helps minimize overlooked symptom domains. Additional clinical tools for assessment are described by Sachs et al., 2003 and accuracy of severity assessments over time can be aided by structured, clinician-administered questionnaires such as the Young Mania Rating Scale (YMRS; Young, Biggs, Ziegler, & Meyer, 1978) for manic symptoms and the Montgomery-Asberg Depression Rating Scale (MADRS; Montgomery, 1979) for depression. Self-report questionnaires for depressive symptoms and suicidal ideation, such as the Beck Depression Inventory-II (BDI- II; Beck, Steer, & Brown, 1996) and the Beck Hopelessness Scale (BHS; Beck, Weissman, Lester, & Trexler, 1974), can also be of use for regular assessments.

Although psychosocial treatments were once relegated to a supportive treatment role, research over the last decade provides support for a powerful role for some of these treatments in the management of bipolar disorder (for review see Miklowitz & Otto, 2006). Moreover, there has been a striking convergence in the strategies of treatment that have been applied in empirical studies of bipolar disorder. In particular, despite differences in theoretical orientation, recent randomized controlled trials of cognitive-behavioral therapy (CBT), family focused therapy (FFT), and interpersonal and social rhythm therapy (IPSRT) share in common (1) psychoeducation that provides patients (and family members) with a model of the nature and course of bipolar disorder, including risk and protective factors such as the role of stress, sleep and lifestyle regularity, and medication adherence; (2) problem-solving and/or communication skills training to reduce the impact of family or external stress; (3) strategies for early detection and intervention for depressive and (hypo)manic episodes, including changes in activities, support levels, and/or intensified pharmacotherapy (Miklowitz et al., 2007; Otto & Miklowitz, 2004).

The empirical support for the use of CBT for bipolar disorder ranges from early studies of the role of brief CBT directed at medication adherence to the validation of more comprehensive interventions aimed at relapse prevention or the treatment of bipolar depression. For example, Cochran (1984) showed that a six-session intervention directed at promoting medication adherence achieved this aim and reduced hospitalization rates over a 6-month follow-up period among patients with bipolar disorder. Perry, Tarrier, Morriss, McCarthy, and Limb (1999) provided 7–12 sessions of CBT focusing on identification of prodromal symptoms and activation of an early-intervention plan (e.g., seeking help from a set of identified health professionals) that was recorded for each patient on a laminated card. This treatment was linked to a significant reduction in the number of manic episodes and to improved social and employment functioning over the next 18 months relative to a routine treatment comparison condition.

Direct transfer of cognitive-behavioral interventions for unipolar depression to bipolar depression was encouraged by a small trial by

Zaretsky, Segal, and Gemar (1999); unipolar and bipolar depression were treated with the same CBT protocol, and both groups achieved similar treatment benefits. More comprehensive application of CBT to bipolar disorder is exemplified by protocols focusing on psychoeducation, cognitive restructuring, regulation of activities and sleep, stress management, interventions for medication adherence, and relapse-prevention strategies. Support for this approach is exemplified by Scott, Garland, and Moorhead (2001) and Lam et al. (2003). For example, Lam et al. (2003) randomized 103 patients to 12 to 18 sessions within the first 6 months and two booster sessions in the second 6 months of care (for a mean of 16 sessions). Participants, outpatients with bipolar disorder, were not in an acute episode when they entered the study, but were characterized by at least two episodes in the last 2 years or three episodes in the last 5 years despite use of mood stabilizers. The results indicated strong protective effects for CBT across 1 year of assessment. Patients in the treatment as usual condition had a relapse rate of 75%, as compared to 43.8% for CBT. Differences were also evident for the number of days in episode status across the year, and trends toward fewer days spent hospitalized due to bipolar disorder, with a mean of 7.3 more days of hospitalization for patients receiving the control treatment.

Evidence for similar efficacy between FFT(e.g., Miklowitz, George, Richards, Simoneau, & Suddath, 2003; Miklowitz & Goldstein, 1997), IPSRT(Frank, Swartz, & Kupfer, 2000; Frank et al., 1997),and CBT (as administered in accordance with this manual) was provided in the context of the very large Systematic Treatment Enhancement Program for Bipolar Disorder (STEP-BD; Miklowitz et al., 2007). The study is distinctive for randomizing a large sample of outpatients with bipolar disorder as well as for examining outcome for three different intensive psychotherapies—CBT, FFT, and IPSRT. The psychosocial treatment in this study is also noteworthy for intervening during the bipolar depressive phase and then continuing interventions with the goal of relapse prevention (as per this manual). These three intensive treatments were compared to a three-session program of supportive and psychoeducational interventions that included a Treatment Contract. The result was that the three intensive treatments were significantly better than the three-session intervention. It is also noteworthy that these psychosocial treatments succeeded where pharmacotherapy did not. That is, in a linked trial, the addition of antidepressants to a mood stabilizer regimen offered no benefit over the addition of placebo (Sachs et al., 2007; see below), whereas, under the same conditions, intensive psychosocial treatments demonstrated significant benefit. These findings help solidify the role of psychosocial treatment in bipolar disorder—succeeding where medications did not.

Overall, evidence from the last decade of study provides converging support for the role of CBT in the management of bipolar disorder. Two limitations should be noted. First, in the CBT protocol offered by Scott et al. (2006), CBT was not more helpful than treatment as usual for individuals who had already had 12 or more mood episodes. Analyses are underway to see whether the current protocol faces the same limitations, but the findings to date do encourage referral of bipolar patients to CBT sooner rather than later in the course of their disorder. A second limitation is that in the formal test of CBT guided by this protocol, the average number of sessions delivered was 14 out of the total 30 sessions of the structured protocol. Nonetheless, consistent with the positive evidence from relapse-prevention applications of CBT for bipolar disorder (e.g., Lam et al., 2003), we anticipate that the current protocol will be applied in a phase-specific way, with emphasis on conducting the first nine sessions during a depressive phase, and then continued or separate application of remaining sessions across the patient's recovery and euthymic period between episodes. In summary, research to date has shown that, with the presumed exclusion of manic episodes where patients may be unable to encode information in a useful way, CBT interventions can offer benefit for the acute depressive, residual symptom, or euthymic phases of the disorder.

The Treatment Manual and the Style of Treatment

Cognitive-behavioral interventions share a focus on teaching patients about the self-perpetuating chains of thoughts, feelings, and behaviors that characterize disorders, and teaching behavioral-change strategies to alter these patterns. Part of this learning is conveyed by verbal instruction in the context of informational interventions or the didactic, self-monitoring, or Socratic methods utilized in cognitive restructuring interventions. Likewise, therapeutic learning is also offered in the wide variety of self-monitoring, role-playing, exposure, activity, and behavioral experiment assignments that are used in CBT protocols. The goal is to make learned information accessible so that patients are able to institute alternative patterns during the moments in life when these alternatives are most needed. To achieve this goal in therapy, learned information needs to be readily accessible. Accessibility is influenced by regular practice of new strategies under relevant conditions. Accessibility is also influenced by the use of strategies that maximize learning and memory cues. For these reasons, there is a consistent focus throughout this manual on the style by which interventions are introduced and practiced.

One formal feature of this treatment manual, similar to other treatment approaches (e.g., Hayes, Strosahl, & Wilson, 1999; Otto 2000), is the active use of stories and metaphors to aid the acquisition of therapeutic concepts. These strategies are used to increase the salience of informational and cognitive restructuring interventions by providing an easy-to-recall format for therapeutic information. Stories are included in specific sessions (e.g., the use of the "coaching story" in Session 2) but are encouraged as a general strategy for change.

To help ensure that CBT is provided in a reliable fashion, this manual details specific interventions to be offered during certain phases of treatment. In addition, a uniform structure for sessions is provided to engender the collaborative, informational, problem-solving focus that characterizes CBT. Likewise, the routine assignment and regular review of home practice procedures as part of the weekly session format ensures a focus on the active, skill-acquisition approach that is at the heart of CBT.

Although sessions are designed to progress in an ordered fashion, with specific content to be reliably delivered at specific treatment points, care is also taken to ensure that cognitive-behavioral analysis is not sacrificed to the goal of uniformity. Specifically in Phase 2, Case Conceptualization Worksheets are used to maintain a flexible modular approach that focuses on a patient's unique problem set rather than forcing all patients into the same "cookie cutter" treatment that has been at the heart of recent criticisms of manualized treatment protocols (see Henin, Otto, &

Reilly-Harrington, 2001). Likewise, consistent attention is given to the style by which interventions are delivered, respecting the diversity with which individuals are prepared to learn. Specifically, the manual directs therapists to use specific strategies to increase the salience of informational interventions and to improve the ease with which skills are remembered and practiced in the relevant moments of a patient's life.

Therapeutic Style

It is important for therapists to adapt a therapeutic style that provides a comfortable emotional fit with the patient. The term "comfortable fit" is hard to describe, but in part describes a collaborative and emotionally rich effort that keeps as its focus the patient's best interests. Although the treatment manual specifies the interventions to be delivered in each session, there is a fair amount of latitude about how these interventions can be delivered. For example, each therapist will need to decide for themselves when a well-toned "hmmm" can replace a full question, or when the exclamation "Ouch!" can be used to replace the phrase, "that sounds like a rather harsh self-criticism." Likewise, each therapist will need to decide how to change, embellish, or replace any of the many existing metaphors used to illustrate treatment concepts. To adhere to this manual, some rich metaphor or vivid discussion should take place, but not necessarily those outlined in a specific session.

It is clear that both the therapist and patient play an active role in treatment. In early sessions particularly, the therapist provides a wealth of new information, guiding the patient toward strategies to be utilized in treatment. However, care should be taken in dosing this information throughout the session, with the therapist remaining attentive to when the patient appears to be eager for additional information, versus when discussion of previously presented information may be the most relevant course. Also, starting in Session 1, effort is placed on helping the patient assume the role of *co-therapist*. This role is important for engendering the active practice of therapy skills and for fully applying the self-care, problem-solving, and well-being skills that comprise the final three stages of treatment. Informational interventions, including the use of instructive metaphors, are part of the attempt to transfer the role of therapist to the patient. The therapist's job is in part to teach the patient how to manage depression and to be an effective cognitive-behavioral therapist for herself. As such, the goal of therapy includes an effort to make the therapist redundant to the patient's own efforts for health.

In all cases, the therapist needs to pay attention to the emotional experience of the patient. Research indicates that dysfunctional cognitions are differentially accessible depending on mood states, with negative moods eliciting more negative cognitions. If the therapist unwittingly avoids emotionally charged ("hot") discussions in session, important opportunities for cognitive restructuring will surely be lost. Emotionally charged discussions also provide therapists with the opportunity to directly model emotional problem-solving skills. This point is so central to the treatment of depression and the process of cognitive restructuring that it deserves additional mention in Chapter 2.

The Role of Medications

This treatment manual is designed for use in conjunction with ongoing pharmacotherapy. The core pharmacotherapy for bipolar disorder is chronic treatment with a mood stabilizer applied singly or in combination with other agents. Lithium is the prototypic mood stabilizer, and has been applied in the United States as a treatment for bipolar disorder for over 30 years. Common agents applied as mood stabilizers also include the anticonvulsants divalproex (Depakote), lamotrigine (Lamictal), and carbamazepine (Tegretol). In recent years, atypical antipsychotics have also shown some promise as mood stabilizers. This class of agents includes aripiprazole (Abilify), olanzapine (Zyprexa), quetiapine (Seroquel), risperidone (Risperdal), and ziprasidone (Geodon). Table 1.1 presents medications that had achieved Federal Drug Administration (FDA) indications for treatment of phases of bipolar disorder as of November 1, 2004.

The pharmacologic treatment of bipolar disorder is associated with significant problems of medication adherence (Keck et al., 1996; Keck et al., 1998). Discontinuation of mood stabilizers brings with it the risk of relapse, particularly when medication is rapidly discontinued (Perlis,

Table 1.1 Agents with FDA Indications for the Treatment of Bipolar Disorder (as of 11/1/2004)

Generic name	Trade name	Acute bipolar depression	Acute bipolar mania	Maintenance treatment of bipolar I disorder
Aripiprazole	Abilify		✓	
Chlorpromazine	Thorazine		✓	
Divalproex	Depakote		✓	
Lamotrigine	Lamictal			✓
Lithium	Eskalith		✓	✓
Olanzapine	Zyprexa		✓	✓
Quetiapine	Seroquel		✓	
Risperidone	Risperdal		✓	
Ziprasidone	Geodon		✓	
Olanzapine/ Fluoxetine combination	Symbyax	✓		

Figure adapted from "Treatment of bipolar disorder: A guide for patients and families," by D. A Kahn, P. E. Keck, R. H. Perlis, M. W. Otto, & R. Ross, 2004, December, *A Postgraduate Medicine Special Report*, pp. 1–108.

Sachs, Lafer, Otto, Faraone, & Rosenbaum, 2002). As noted, brief psychosocial treatment has been successfully applied to the problem of adherence and has been found to improve adherence and the course of bipolar disorder (Cochran, 1984). However, psychosocial treatment can also play a much broader role in the management of bipolar disorder.

Use of antidepressants in combination with mood stabilizers is an especially common strategy (Keck, Perlis, Otto, Carpenter, Docherty, & Ross, 2004), but a number of recent studies have called into question the utility of this approach. For example, Nemeroff et al. (2001) examined the combination of the antidepressants pareoxetine and imipramine as adjunctive treatments to ongoing lithium therapy. Outpatients with bipolar depression who had been treated with lithium for at least 6 weeks were studied. Results indicated no significant benefit for the addition of either of these antidepressants, at least for patients who had adequate lithium levels. A similar absence of efficacy for adjunctive antidepressant treatment was also evident in a large double-blind, placebo-controlled examination of the efficacy of antidepressant treatment (either bupropion or paroxetine) versus placebo as adjunctive interventions to ongoing treatment with mood stabilizers (lithium, valproate, carbamazepine, or other FDA-approved antimanic agents) (Sachs et al., 2007). This very large study was conducted at centers across the United States, and patients with bipolar I or II disorder were treated for up to 26 weeks. No significant differences were found between patients who received a mood stabilizer plus an antidepressant and those who received a mood stabilizer plus placebo in terms of recovery from depression. Together, the studies by Sachs et al. (2007) and Nemeroff et al. (2001) raise serious questions about the efficacy of using antidepressants to relieve bipolar depression. It is especially noteworthy that it in the absence of significant beneficial effects for antidepressants (Sachs et al., 2007), significant benefit was found for psychosocial treatment (CBT, FFT, and IPSRT) for bipolar depression in the same cohort of patients (Miklowitz et al., 2007).

Use of the Patient Workbook

In addition to this guide, there is a corresponding workbook available for patients. The workbook contains psychoeducational information that the patient can refer to in between sessions to reinforce what is learned during treatment. It also contains worksheets and forms for use during in-session exercises, as well as for completing at-home assignments. Be sure to instruct the patient to bring the workbook to every meeting.

Chapter 2 | *Overview of Treatment Structure and Strategies*

Phases of Treatment

This cognitive-behavioral therapy (CBT) program is organized around the delivery of 30 sessions (21 weekly and 9 biweekly) for amelioration of an acute depressive episode and training in relapse prevention. Treatment proceeds in four formal phases:

1. Depression-focus phase (9 sessions)

2. Treatment-contract phase (4 sessions)

3. Problem-list phase (13 sessions)

4. Well-being phase (4 sessions)

In each phase, similar cognitive-behavioral procedures are utilized, but the targets and style of therapy shift according to the treatment phase.

Depression-Focus Phase (Phase 1)

The first nine sessions of treatment are aimed exclusively at amelioration of the patient's depression. Treatment emphasizes informational interventions, cognitive restructuring, and activity assignments. Initial interventions are devoted to orienting the patient toward a cognitive-behavioral perspective and engaging the patient in the treatment process. In the first session, emphasis is placed on helping the patient adopt a "therapeutic perspective" toward his own care. This is done to enlist the patient as a co-therapist on the case and is a first step toward helping the patient develop the sense of benevolent self-evaluation and guidance that is at the heart of cognitive restructuring efforts. Early work on the "therapeutic perspective" provides a natural segue to self-monitoring that in turn provides the basis for later cognitive restructuring interventions. Cognitive restructuring is aimed at correcting the distorted and dysfunctional evaluations that characterize depression. At the same time, activity assignments are used to help return the patient to the adaptive behaviors and pleasant events that can engender and sustain improvements in mood.

Treatment-Contract Phase (Phase 2)

This phase of treatment consists of three sessions of treatment devoted to completion of the Treatment Contract and delineation of topics for the next phase of treatment, and one session educating the patient about hyperpositive thinking. The main therapeutic tool of this stage is completion of the Treatment Contract, which can be found in the patient workbook. Due to the need for a more intensive focus on depression at the outset, the Treatment Contract is not reviewed until this stage of treatment. Also, it is advantageous to focus on the therapy contract once a good therapeutic alliance has been made, the patient has a positive and hopeful attitude toward therapy, and, hopefully, periods of euthymia have been reestablished. It is under these conditions that rapid progression through the therapy contract can be achieved. During the contracting stage of treatment, involvement of the family is encouraged.

Problem-List Phase (Phase 3)

The third phase of treatment utilizes a modular design to target problem areas of greatest concern to the patient and the therapist. This includes continued intensive treatment targeting depression, attention to comorbid anxiety disorders if present, and attention to specific problem areas by, for example, developing assertiveness or communication skills that may aid the patient in buffering the effects of stress and preventing future mood episodes.

Case Conceptualization Worksheets (see Chapter 16) are used during this phase of treatment to guide the relevant modules to be used in remaining treatment sessions. This manual includes six modules that address the following topics:

- Problem solving

- Social skills

- Anxiety

- Relaxation and breathing training

- Anger management

- Extreme emotions

For these comorbid conditions, the goal is not to provide full treatment, but rather to provide a range of relevant skills to decrease distress and reduce the contribution of these conditions to depressive and manic symptoms.

Well-Being Phase (Phase 4)

Well-being therapy (Fava, Rafanelli, Cazzaro, Conti, & Grandi, 1998; Fava & Ruini, 2003) is a clinical approach that attends to the metaphorical "other side of the coin" from traditional CBT. That is, instead of focusing primary attention on the reduction of symptoms, well-being therapy emphasizes maximization of periods of well-being. This feature makes it an ideal approach for the final stage of treatment where gains are to be solidified and extended. There is evidence that well-being therapy is a useful strategy for dealing with residual symptoms of depression (see Fava et al., 1998). Likewise, its focus on extending periods of well-being and utilizing cognitive-behavioral skills for subsyndromal symptoms makes it an ideal relapse-prevention strategy. In well-being therapy, periods of well-being are monitored and discussed. Corresponding clinical interventions are designed to remove cognitive and behavioral habits and strategies that interfere with the attainment or maintenance of well-being. Of course, the clinical interventions for removing blocks to well-being may well be identical to the ones that would be applied under a traditional CBT approach. However, they are couched under the broader umbrella of improving quality of life.

The Structure of Sessions

Each session is formulated into a problem-solving format that includes (a) a review of the patient's mood over the past week, (b) a review of the previous week's learning, including homework, (c) the formulation of an agenda for the session and completion of the agenda with attention to in-session rehearsal of concepts, (d) a summary of the session content, and (e) assignment of home practice. This format maintains a consistent focus on the step-by-step, goal-oriented, skill-acquisition approach that is at the heart of this treatment.

Mood Chart Review

Sessions typically begin with a "mood check." This is best done by reviewing the patient's completed Mood Chart. The Mood Chart is a recommended part of this program; formal introduction to charting in the context of CBT occurs in Session 2 (also see Chapter 2 of the workbook). Mood charting provides a systematic assessment of daily changes in mood, sleep patterns, and medication compliance, as well as a report on daily stressors. Ideally, by viewing the patient's Mood Chart, you will get a rapid snapshot of the past week. In this way, you can quickly get a sense of problem areas and add them to the agenda for discussion. Many patients also find that presenting the Mood Chart to their therapist saves time in the session for issues of greatest importance to them. Rather than a lengthy dialogue recapping mood changes and weekly events, the Mood Chart allows a quick transition to specific topics. Of course, this strategy is helpful only if the patient complies with completion of the Mood Chart. Reviewing the Mood Chart at the beginning of each session tends to improve compliance. More information on compliance can be found at the end of the chapter.

Homework Review

The previous week's home practice is also reviewed at the start of each session. This process provides continuity between sessions and underscores that the therapist and the patient are working toward a set of goals for which home practice is important. In particular, homework review includes a brief summary of some of the content of the previous session, linking that content to home practice.

Because homework review naturally bridges the gap between the last session's content and the assigned work, it provides patients with an opportunity to examine how well they are making use of session material. At times, patients will be surprised at how poorly they recall the previous session's content, or they may think of the therapy hour as the primary time where therapeutic work is done. Homework review helps maintain the focus on the expectation that the therapy hour is a time to conceptualize and rehearse the change process, but that much of the work to reach goals occurs between sessions.

Agenda Setting

Review of home practice also provides a natural segue into a discussion of successes or difficulties with session content, and this information can be integrated into the setting of agenda for the current session. The agenda should include items from the manual as well as discussion of any concerns, new problems, or questions raised by the patient. In general, the patient's concerns will be scheduled early in the agenda, and the manual-driven targets for the session will be discussed, whenever possible, in relation to areas of difficulty noted by the patient. For example, difficulties with an activity assignment (from Session 3) may be used as an example for the next stage of cognitive restructuring (in Session 4).

Session Summary

Each session should include a summary of topics covered in that session. In providing a review of core concepts, it is important for the therapist to keep in mind the memory and concentration-disrupting effects of depression. Moreover, session content frequently elicits strong and sometimes distracting emotions in the patient, which can impact memory for session content. Review of session content provides an opportunity to consolidate information for the patient. In providing this consolidation, it is important to include the patient in the process. For example, the therapist may ask the patient to repeat in his own words some of the concepts he wants to remember from the session.

Homework Assignments

Sessions should conclude with the assignment of homework (for some patients, the term "home practice" may be more acceptable and more accurate than "homework"). This assignment should flow naturally from the summary of session content (e.g., *"Given what we covered today, it will be important for you to practice this new skill during the week and see how it works for you"*). Home practice should not be given without some "troubleshooting" of the difficulties or problems the patient may have implementing the homework, in terms of either scheduling or emotional obstacles. Finally, the therapist should close by reminding the patient that the goal of home practice is learning, not having to do something "perfectly." It is the learning through difficulties with an assignment that sometimes leads to an especially productive follow-up session.

Recording Sessions

As noted, the home practice assignments maintain the expectation that much of the work to reach goals occurs between sessions; the therapy hour is a time to conceptualize and rehearse the change process. Regular tape recording of the session content is encouraged for this reason. Starting in Session 1, the patient is encouraged to allow tape recording of the session and to listen to the tape before the next session. This procedure allows a patient to effectively double the information derived from any session. Recording of sessions is encouraged primarily during the first eight sessions of treatment, when greater amounts of didactic information are presented and skills are rehearsed for the first time. Over time, recording of sessions should decrease.

Of course, recording of sessions for patient review is fully up to the patient. Many patients may be reluctant to hear their voice on tape. The therapist should encourage the taping, but not be insistent. Taping should end whenever patient and therapist agree that the additional information gained is not substantial or is diminished by patient concerns.

Treatment Elements

Informational Interventions

Informational components are designed to provide the patient with a model of the disorder, a rationale for treatment procedures, and a guide for the patient's collaborative treatment efforts. In the early stages of treatment, attention is devoted to characterizing elements of the disorder for the patient, and mobilizing the patient's efforts at change. This process involves teaching individuals the cognitive-behavioral model of the interplay between thoughts, feelings, and behaviors. The patient is asked to then complement this didactic information by observing his own experiences, testing the model, and identifying for himself the role of thoughts in influencing mood. Informational interventions are also used to define strategies for change (e.g., the purpose and rationale behind homework assignments) and to provide "signposts" for the change process (interim signs of progress).

Cognitive Restructuring

Cognitive restructuring (CR) focuses directly on the modification of dysfunctional and depressogenic cognitions and core beliefs during the acute depression phase, and then later focuses on the role of hyperpositive thoughts, which, in addition to being a symptom of (hypo)mania, may serve as a causal or maintaining factor for this mood phase. Later, in the Problem List Phase, cognitive restructuring interventions are applied to the management of comorbid conditions.

Cognitive restructuring is based on the premise that feelings and behaviors are influenced by one's perception of events. For CR, thoughts are treated as hypotheses, and emphasis is placed on the development of more accurate thinking patterns. No attempt is made to have patients think "happy thoughts." Instead, the focus is on helping patients maximize adaptive and realistic patterns of thinking. Cognitive restructuring strategies include guided discussions, Socratic questioning, and self-monitoring, that may or may not be enhanced by story heuristics such as the coaching story in Session 2. In addition, cognitive change is also aided significantly by "behavioral experiment" procedures. In a behavioral experiment, programmed experiences are used to test the validity of specific beliefs. Presumably, patients observe their performance and the outcome of events in such situations and abstract more adaptive expectations and rules for future exposures. The use of behavioral experiments underscores the reality that cognitive change does not need to rely on verbal argument. Instead, behavioral experiments use specific observations of reality to help individuals bring their cognitions in line with actual outcomes.

In the present treatment, CR interventions are introduced after clarification of the status of thoughts, whereby the patient is reminded that thoughts are behaviors. Under ideal conditions, thoughts are tools for adaptive living. However, it is a mistake to pay more attention to thoughts than to actual events in life, or to let thoughts inaccurately color the perception of events. Overall, the patient is taught that thoughts are behaviors that should not be considered as *correct or incorrect* so much as they should be evaluated as *useful or not*. One of the goals of CR is to eliminate reliance on maladaptive cognitions and to guide the patient to useful alternatives.

Although these categories are far from distinct, cognitive restructuring can attend to any of three interrelated targets for change: (1) the emotional tone of self-talk, (2) distortions in the interpretation of events, and (3) the development of more useful cognitive skills. It is up to the clinician, especially in latter treatment sessions, to determine which of these elements to emphasize the most in the context of CR interventions.

Attention to the emotional tone of self-talk receives initial attention in Session 1. In this session, emphasis is placed on the adoption of therapeutic empathy and the use of a reasonable tone for self-talk. Additional attention is placed on this style at the end of Session 2, with review of the coaching story. The goal of these interventions is to replace punitive, harsh, or mocking self-talk with supportive and adaptive self-guidance. Accordingly, at any point throughout treatment, it is appropriate to modify the tone of cognitions.

Cognitive restructuring, which evaluates the accuracy of thoughts, receives formal attention in Session 3 and thereafter. For these interventions, the patient is taught to evaluate the accuracy of thoughts, using information on common cognitive distortions in conjunction with regular self-monitoring. The goal is to help the patient inhibit automatic cognitive responses to events and to select alternative, accurate explanations.

Attention to the elimination of distortions and the negative tone of cognitions is complemented by interventions to increase adaptive self-talk. These interventions are based on the notion that attempts to decrease maladaptive behavior do not necessarily increase adaptive habits. Interventions to aid adaptive self-talk are initiated in the context of the coaching story and receive additional attention as part of CR and problem-solving skills.

To complete CR exercises, patients are asked to be aware of their emotions in the moment, and upon detecting an emotional change, to examine both the external situation ("What is going on?") and their internal environment ("What have I been saying to myself?"). Ideally, this process is completed with a sense of empathy toward oneself: "I am feeling bad; how can I understand what is going on?" These questions guide the patient toward a specific style of self-examination. Emotions are respected for what they are, and self-punitive responses to emotions are replaced with more adaptive alternatives (regardless of whether these alternatives involve cognitive restructuring, overt problem solving, or acceptance of a negative event).

Access to relevant emotions and the "hot" cognitions that may accompany these emotions is aided by the self-monitoring and review of problematic events and emotions that is a part of standard CBT. It is important for therapists to utilize these emotional opportunities by applying manualized interventions to the emotions at hand. For example, didactic information about cognitive restructuring should be delivered in relation to the patient's emotional state in the session, not in spite of it. However, learning in the context of "hot" emotions can be derailed by a patient's reluctance to experience these emotions. The therapist's comfort with the patient's emotions, and the delivery of appropriate empathy occurring in conjunction with a problem-solving approach, provides a model for the skills to be acquired by the patient. This essential modeling should be thought of as a central feature of CBT.

Activity Assignments

Activity assignments are utilized in conjunction with CR with the goals of returning depressed patients to pleasant and rewarding activities as well as providing a balance of activities to aid mood stability once euthymia is achieved. Activity scheduling is initiated with self-monitoring of current activities and is followed by the review and subsequent assignment of potentially pleasant events from a list of possibilities. Cognitive restructuring plays a crucial role in preparing patients for adaptively approaching and interpreting their responses to activity assignments. Activity assignments are also used as buffers against stress by helping patients adopt a regular schedule with rewarding breaks. Self-monitoring of this schedule provides a context for examining self-reinforcement and ensuring adaptive cognitive responses to the true level of activity and achievements. In addition, during later phases of treatment, an activity schedule can provide clues that a mood episode may be emerging. For example, if a patient recognizes that he is having difficulty carrying out activities (or in the case of a hypomanic phase, activities have greatly increased), the therapist can use this information as part of an early intervention program.

The first step in a program of activity assignments is to assess, collaboratively with the patient, the current level of activity and its impact on the patient. As will be clear from the following examples, activity assignment exercises provide excellent opportunities for CR. In fact, evaluation of a patient's cognitions about an assignment, particularly regarding the expected level of performance, is a standard component of activity assignments. Exemplified in the section that follows are select stages of activity monitoring that illustrate the combination of cognitive and activity interventions. Particular attention is devoted to the range of ways that cognitive interventions may be employed.

We also exemplify the use of "behavioral experiments" either in the context of role-play situations or home assignments, or provide the patient with the opportunity to examine the accuracy of his thoughts while helping him rehearse life situations relevant to activity assignments.

Introducing Activity Assignments

The first step in developing an activity chart is to help the patient consider some of the activities that he used to enjoy or believes are important. This process is aided by the activity assignments in the patient workbook, which are designed to help patients consider relevant domains for rewarding activities. Further help in generating potential rewarding activities is provided by the Pleasant Events list in the workbook.

After compiling a list of proposed activities, the therapist should assist the patient in identifying a starting point. Frequently patients want to begin with activities that are guilt-based, based on a sense of being "behind" in the basic activities of daily living. It is important to encourage an activity plan that is well rounded, including activities from a range of categories including social, recreational, exercise/sport, hobby, relationship, and work-related activities, rather than simply the guilt-inducing activities that have been long avoided by the patient. Consider the following case vignette, where P represents the patient and T represents the therapist:

Case Vignette

P: I am so overwhelmed by all the work I need to do around the house. My place is a mess. I know I need to do some things around the house. But, I do not know where to start.

T: It sounds overwhelming. It might be helpful if we come up with a plan to help you accomplish the tasks you want to get done around the house.

P: Well, I haven't had a regular schedule for household tasks in over 6 months. As a result I have fallen so far behind that I will never catch up. In fact, because there is so much to do it makes it even harder for me to get motivated to do it.

T: Well, it is important that you don't try to tackle everything at once. Let's try to devise a plan together that is gradual so that you don't feel so overwhelmed, but that allows you begin to do some of the things you've been wanting to do.

P: Sounds OK, but to be honest I am not sure I am going to have the energy to do much.

T: Well, that is another reason why it is important that you begin to do things gradually. I think that if we put a plan in place, you might find the structure is helpful. Let's consider it an experiment. I bet that when you begin to do some of the things you have been putting off, you are going to feel better about yourself and the situation.

P: I sure hope so.

T: Before we come up with a specific plan, it is important for me to get some idea of the activities you are currently doing on a daily basis.

P: As I told you, I am doing very little. I spend most of my day sleeping or laying in bed thinking about what I am not doing.

T: Regardless of what you are doing, I would like you to spend the next week using the Weekly Activity Schedule in your workbook to monitor what you do on a daily basis. Your descriptions can be very brief. For example, you may write "sat in chair, drank coffee, and watched TV."

P: OK. I'll give it a try.

Frequently, the patient reports a higher level of activity than he expected. It is important to point this out and use this information to challenge some of the patient's original comments like "I can't get anything done" or "I don't do anything at all anymore." Baseline information is also important for gauging actual activity and improvement in activity level.

For patients in the depressed phase, a poorly designed activity assignment may result in failure and confirmation from the patient of his thoughts that "I can't get anything right" or "I am stupid." It may be more reasonable to choose only one task and break it into smaller steps. Assess this closely with each patient. Over successive weeks of treatment, you will continue to add activities with increasing complexity and time commitment. It is important to incorporate pleasant events (e.g., social contact, hobbies) in addition to mastery-based tasks (e.g., household chores) to the patient's activity plan.

Because it is common for individuals to focus more on the completion of a task rather than its initiation, it is important to help the patient plan the initiation of the task (day, time of day, helpful cues, etc.), and to help the patient break tasks/activities into component steps. These component steps increase the opportunity for completion and also provide targets for incremental success. Consider the following case vignette:

Case Vignette

T: Last session you said that you feel overwhelmed by all the tasks you were not performing on a regular basis. Nonetheless, when we set up this plan, it is important that we get you back into attempting these tasks gradually. Last session you generated a pretty long list of chores around the house that you feel need to be done. Can you pick just a few of these to get started?

P: It is hard to do that. They are all necessary.

T: How about starting with a few activities that are the least time consuming?

P: In that case, maybe I can start with sweeping the porch every few days, watering the plants in the garden once a day, washing my dishes every day, and grocery shopping a couple times a week so I have food in the house.

T: How about picking only two of those activities this week and adding one that is a bit more enjoyable from your activities list?

Refer the patient back to the Activity Schedule and help him plan and choose particular times for completing each activity. It is crucial to assist the patient in identifying potential problems in attempting the task. Likewise, you should use a problem-solving approach to enhance the likelihood that the patient will attempt the assigned task. Especially at first, emphasis should be placed on attempting rather than completing a task.

Case Vignette

T: When might be the best times each day to complete these activities?

P: I don't know. Mornings aren't good. I am so depressed and sleepy in the mornings.

T: Is there a particular time of the day that you typically feel your best?

P: Yes, late afternoon.

T: That may be the best time for you to do these activities, if possible. As we add more activities later it won't be possible to cram them all into the late afternoon, but for now let's try to increase the chances that you will feel like attempting these activities by performing them at a time when you are likely to feel your best. If it sounds OK to you, go ahead and write in your plan on the activity schedule.

Stepwise Goal Attainment

An additional component of problem solving is training in stepwise goal attainment. For larger or longer-term goals, it may be necessary to help patients structure the logical increments to goal attainment. For example, if a patient has a goal to buy and drive a new car, initial goals may be to save a certain amount of money per week and/or search the Internet to identify reasonable car prices. Later goals may include shopping for a car, examining financing options, etc. A Long-Term Goal Sheet (stair-step diagram) is provided in Chapter 8 of the workbook (a copy for your reference is provided in the appendix). Instruct the patient to use this sheet if relevant for his progress.

A central component of the therapist's job in CBT is to educate the patient about maladaptive patterns and adaptive alternatives, program these changes, and assign relevant home practice to help the patient execute these changes. Because poor compliance with homework is associated with poorer outcome, CBT therapists should make every effort to aid the patient with achieving compliance with home-practice procedures.

When faced by noncompliance, behavior therapists should evaluate whether the desired setting conditions for the assignment were met. These setting conditions represent some of the conditions under which homework compliance can be facilitated.

1. The patient understands the rationale for this intervention and the potential gains that may be achieved.

2. The patient has the component skills to apply this intervention. That is, the skill involved in the assignment is a reasonable increment given the patient's current abilities.

3. The patient rehearsed an intervention of this kind in session before being asked to do it out of the session.

4. Fears and dysfunctional expectations associated with the assignment have been examined.

5. Potential blocks to homework compliance have been examined in a problem-solving format.

6. The patient has sufficient cues to *remember* to apply the assignment.

7. The patient is able to recognize the conditions under which the home practice should be completed.

8. The patient is an active participant in the assignment.

Strategies to help maximize these setting conditions are described in the following sections.

Motivation for Completing Assignments

An occasional reason for poor adherence is that the assignment was inadequately linked with the patient's goals. Patients should be told why a specific intervention is being given and provided with at least minimal expectations of the benefits of the home practice. Giving the patient "signposts" for change may further enhance motivation. That is, patients should be provided with examples of what they should experience (e.g., feel, say, and think) during the assignment if it is going well. Consider the following case vignette.

T: Because you are preparing to approach this problem with your brother-in-law differently, what do you think you may feel when you try the response we picked today?

P: I think I will feel odd, and may be kind of worried.

T: Exactly! I think that when you start to do something differently from what you have been doing during the last several months, you will feel odd. You are no longer doing the expected; you are out of the "rut." And because you are doing something that is different from the old habit, you may feel kind of odd and kind of anxious. In fact, I would take that as a sign that you are on track. If you feel odd and anxious when interacting with your brother-in-law, this may be the very sign that you are on track with the new alternatives we discussed.

Manageable Increments Between Skills

A good strategy for success is to send a patient out to complete a home practice assignment only after that assignment has been rehearsed in session (either through a role-play or imaginal completion of the exercise). Likewise, if the patient returns to a session stating that an assignment was too hard, the therapist should rehearse component elements in session. In this case, the therapist may reassign only an element of the previous week's homework to help ensure that the assignment is manageable.

Assessment and Management of Fears and Dysfunctional Expectations

Homework assignments provide an excellent opportunity for cognitive restructuring. When assigning homework, ask whether the patient expects to have any difficulties with the assignment. Help the patient problem solve by asking him to identify "the hardest aspect of the assignment." Management of presumed or actual difficulties with an assignment provides you with the opportunity to further exemplify problem-solving strategies and/or cognitive restructuring.

Difficulties "Remembering" the Assignment

Patients may have poor compliance simply because it is difficult to remember an intervention during the week between the sessions. In addition to the use of vivid examples and stories, you may want to have the patient audio record the session and then listen to the recording during the week mid-way between scheduled sessions. Alternatively, you may write out (or have the patient write out) specific assignments. The use of colored stick-on-dots available at office supply stores can also be helpful. Provide the patient with the stickers and instruct him to place them in locations where he will see them several times a day (e.g., on his telephone, bathroom mirror, and door knobs) Explain that the dots represent the things discussed in that week's therapy session and when the patient sees them, he will be reminded of his homework assignment.

Rehearsals

To help the patient apply interventions, it is helpful to rehearse them under relevant conditions. For example, it makes more sense to rehearse an anxiety-management skill when the patient is anxious rather than relaxed. Whenever possible, use role-plays to identify the relevant internal (mood) or external (people or places) cues for application of a new skill. By rehearsing the new skill (e.g., assertiveness) in response to relevant role-played cues (e.g., a demanding person), the patient can be more optimally prepared to apply this skill out of the session.

Using Reminder Cues

One way to prepare the patient to try alternative skills is to provide him with a metaphor of the change process. One of our favorite metaphors within Action and Commitment Therapy (Hayes et al., 1999) concerns a patient's perspective when entering treatment. The metaphor utilizes the image of an individual who has fallen in a hole and is desperately trying to get out. In trying to get out, this person is using the tool that is at hand, a shovel. Regardless of whether the patient digs fast or slower, with big shovelfuls or small, he will still be in the hole, because the tool being used is for digging—not for getting out of the hole. The metaphor next introduces the idea of a ladder as an alternative to continuing to dig with the shovel (existing habits). In order to use the ladder, however, one has to let go of the shovel. Releasing the shovel is often the hardest part.

As detailed in Otto (2000), this metaphor provides the patient with a rationale for understanding that old habits are often difficult to "put down," and likewise that new and useful alternatives may initially feel uncomfortable. In addition, the shovel and ladder metaphor provides useful visual cues that can be extended to homework assignments. When maladaptive patterns are identified, these patterns and cues for these patterns can be written on the shovel side of the card. Cues linked with collaboratively identified alternative responses are written on the ladder side of the card. The patient is then given the card as a reminder of the situations where new skills/alternative responses are to be applied. Patients who like the "shovel/ladder" metaphor are frequently pleased by this method of providing a brief, written, characterization of session content and upcoming challenges.

Involving the Patient as Co-Therapist

In every case, efforts should be made to involve the patient in the decision of what sort of home practice is relevant. Even when specific assignments are scripted for early sessions, you should discuss the assignment with the patient, asking whether the homework seems relevant or whether it should be altered in some way to make it more consistent with the patient's goals. If a patient initially refuses an assignment or is pessimistic, restate the goals of the assignment and problem solve for alternative methods of achieving the therapeutic goal. In all cases, you have the freedom to alter the form of an assignment to aid the patient with compliance and enhance the overall goal of skill acquisition.

Troubleshooting Medication Compliance

Given the potential costs of medication discontinuation, particularly rapid medication discontinuation, in bipolar disorder (Perlis et al., 2002), it is crucial for the CBT therapist to help manage medication adherence. Regular review of the patient's adherence to the medication regimen should be part of the review of progress and assignments that starts each session. If difficulties with medication adherence are identified, the therapeutic discussion shifts to identification of specific obstacles to adherence. Common obstacles associated with low adherence include medication side effects, remittance of symptoms that may suggest to the patient a decreased need for medications, an unsupportive social network, conflicts between medication scheduling and personal time demands, and beliefs about being "overdependent" on medications. Identified obstacles can then be examined as part of the CR and problem-solving interventions that are a regular part of treatment. Following are several case vignettes that highlight clinical issues associated with medication compliance.

Case Vignette 1

The patient is a 34-year-old, single woman who suffers from rapid-cycling bipolar disorder and bulimia. Most psychiatric medications had done little to curtail her racing thoughts and hypomanic behavior. However, she began taking a new medication regime that showed promise but could cause weight gain. Given her long-standing history of bulimia, she was quite reluctant to take medication that may exacerbate one of these problems.

T: So your psychiatrist put you on some new medications.

P: Yeah, whatever, as if these are going to work. I've tried so many now, I feel like a guinea pig.

T: You have tried a lot. I can understand that you feel upset that you've tried so many, and I wish that the first ones worked better. Have you started taking these new ones?

P: Well, I started today. I don't know. Why bother?

T: If we look back at your history of medication trials, it is pretty apparent that they did not work for individual reasons. One caused you to become nauseous, one gave you a rash, and the other two didn't seem to make much of a difference. If we examine each one individually, it doesn't seem that all medications are completely ineffectual. I hope you can at least give these a try.

P: I will. I promised my doctor that I would give it 2 weeks.

> *The patient remained compliant with her medications, but she began to gain weight. Weight gain was especially significant as this patient had a history of bulimia and anorexia in her past. We discussed compliance within the context of her eating disorder history.*

P: I know I'm fat. I mean look at me! (She was actually underweight for her size.) I don't think I can take this medication anymore. I'm not going to let myself get fatter! It's not worth it! I'd rather be skinny.

T: How much weight have you gained?

P: I don't know, 3 or 4 pounds. I just know I'm fat.

T: But you are much less racy, and your thoughts are under your control. You are also sleeping more regularly. I would hate to lose these benefits. We have to find the middle ground here. How can you keep on taking medication that finally works, while not gaining weight, which would make you stop it? Are you eating more?

P: No, I keep a daily food log for my nutritionist. I think I'm eating just as much as before.

T: What about exercise?

P: Well, I've kinda stopped going to the gym. I just don't have the time, and I don't care about going.

T: Do you think that you might have gained some weight because you are not as active?

P: That might be it. I mean I haven't been to the gym since I left your office last week.

T: I would suggest getting you back into some sort of regular exercise plan. Not only would you lose some weight, or at least maintain the weight you are at, but it would also provide you with some structure and some relief from your stress. How about we look at where you can bring exercise back into your daily plan?

With some planning, the patient was able to return to a regular routine of exercise. She did not gain any more weight, and she was able to feel better about herself and her medication regime.

Case Vignette 2

The patient is a 21-year-old male with a recent onset of bipolar I, manic. After a moderately destructive manic episode, he was hospitalized and prescribed neuroleptic medication. He had particular concerns about feeling emotionless and wanted to go off of his medication temporarily, to make himself feel high again.

P: So they put me on these meds which are supposed to make my mood stable. I don't know. It makes me feel like I have no mood at all, like a zombie.

T: I know what you mean. When people who have been manic go on a mood stabilizing medication for the first time, they often feel as if their emotions are nonexistent.

P: Exactly! It's like I don't have any feelings.

T: But you still have feelings. They are not as extreme now, so it feels different. Often after you have been to the extremes of your emotions like you were during your manic episode, emotions that are less intense feel dull. Sometimes you might even feel lifeless.

P: Really? I don't know. Sometimes I think that I should just go off my meds, just for a little while, so that I can feel that high again. I liked that intensity.

T: Although it might be more intense, you unfortunately end up losing control over your feelings.

P: Tell me about it. I messed up my relationship with my girlfriend. I said some things that were nasty. But maybe I can just go off of them on the weekends. This way, I can be up for when my friends and I go out. I like going out on the weekends. Who wants to hang out with a doorknob?

T: Playing around with your medication like that is tricky. A mood stabilizer has to build up in your system, and you need a certain level in your blood for it to work. If you stop your medication on the weekends, you might end up losing control again.

P: My friends always tell me that they like me because I'm funny and I make people laugh. I don't feel up with these meds.
(Here may be an ideal place to address cognitions and perceptions about self that may be interfering with medication compliance.)

T: Is it possible that concerns with your medication may have something to do with the way you perceive yourself?

P: You think so?

T: I don't think a mood stabilizer is going to take away your personality. It may seem to you that you are less funny, but I think it would be good to ask your friends if that is really the case when you are on your meds.

P: I bet they will say I am less fun now.

T: And what if they do say that? What is so bad about being less funny than usual?

P: Well, I guess nothing really. Except that my friends might not like being with me as much.

T: You and I discussed previously that your friends have a hard time being around you when you are elevated.

P: Oh, I know! I remember last time I would say something that I thought was funny, but then nobody would laugh, and then I would start swearing at them. These were my best friends and here I was cursing at them in a club. They wouldn't talk to me for a long time after that. I think you might be right.

T: But you also have a fear that your personality that you had before is gone now. I think that before you make that assumption, you should check it out with your friends.

P: You mean ask them?

T: Yeah. I think it would make sense to ask them how much you have changed for the better or worse before you make a decision to stop your medication. That is a big risk, and it would make sense to go slowly with any decision about your medication.

P: Okay, I think I will ask them. I guess I might not be the best judge of my moods and personality right now.

Case Vignette 3

The patient is a 24-year-old woman with a 2-year history of bipolar disorder. She has had two manic episodes followed rather quickly by depressive episodes. She has been consistently noncompliant with her medication. She has come in after another manic episode that required a long hospitalization.

T: So, how are we going to help you take your medications?

P: I just forget, you know? It's not like I haven't heard all this before. I'm going to nod my head and agree that it's important and then I'm going to go home and put my pills in my medicine cabinet and then forget about them.

T: Why do you think that you forget to take your meds?

P: I don't know, maybe it's subconscious or something. I don't want to think that these meds are controlling me. So, maybe I don't take them to avoid reality.

T: Well, then it seems that we have two issues happening here. One is learning some strategies to help you remember to take your meds on a regular basis. The other is your sense of what it means to be diagnosed with bipolar disorder. I think that both are important areas to address to help you take your medication more regularly.

P: (nods)

T: Let's consider some strategies to help you take your medication regularly. Is there any other place that you can keep your medication so that you will be sure to take them? It seems that the medicine cabinet is not a good place, because it keeps it hidden from view.

P: I guess I could put it on my nightstand by my bed. I always have a glass of water there so it would be convenient.

T: Now what about a reminder somewhere else in your home to make sure that you take the medication?

P: Yeah, I often leave the house and think, "Oops, I forgot again."

T: How about a written reminder by your door? Maybe writing something simple like, "Meds" and taping it to your door. This would serve as a cue to remind yourself to take your medication before you head out the door.

P: I could do that, but I would take it down if I have company. No way would I leave something like that up, or even have my medications out there in the open for someone to see them.

T: In that event, you might leave a reminder to put the sign back up. Your concerns about what other people might think about you taking medication brings up the other point we discussed—the way you perceive your illness.

P: I hate that word, "illness!" Why does everyone say that to me? I mean, I hate the fact that I'm going to need a pill to make me normal.

T: I know. Many people with bipolar disorder hate taking a pill to control their mood. We're taught that we should always be in control of our emotions. But many people with chronic illnesses like high blood pressure and diabetes also hate taking medication, and they also hate the fact that something inside of them feels uncontrollable.

P: I never made the connection with physical illnesses. That makes sense, but I'm not going to be telling everyone that I'm mentally ill.

T: You have the right to tell who you want, when you want.

P: I know. I also need to start telling myself that many people take medications every day to treat their problems. Mine is no different.

T: I'm not glossing over your experience. It is hard to take medication on a regular basis. But the more you take your medications, the more control you will have. Let's try it for this week and see what happens. I hope you're not nodding your head like the other times.

P: No, this time is different.

T: How about if we check in over the phone later in the week to see how it is going?

P: I'll call you later this week and let you know how things are going.

T: It's a deal.

Treatment Phase 1

Chapter 3

Session 1: Introduction

(Corresponds to chapter 1 of the workbook)

Materials Needed

- Self-Care Worksheet for Suicidal Thoughts
- Audio recorder (optional)

Outline

- Review confidentiality policy and patient's previous treatments
- Introduce a model for conceptualizing depression
- Introduce the notion of biased thinking
- Discuss the role of cognitions in depression
- Discuss depression's effect on activity levels
- Review CBT model of depression
- Discuss the importance of self-care
- Have the patient complete the Self-Care Worksheet for Suicidal Thoughts and contract for safety
- Assign homework
- Close with evaluations of the session and homework

The purpose of the first session of treatment is to orient the patient to the assumptions and methods of cognitive-behavioral therapy (CBT) for depression, and initiate treatment of self-depreciating reactions to depression symptoms (i.e., depression about depression). In this session, the patient is provided with a model of depression, its maintenance, and its treatment. Attention is placed on helping the patient identify symptoms as part of a syndrome and inhibit self-blame or other dysfunctional cognitive reactions to the disorder. These interventions also provide the framework for helping the patient mobilize a therapeutic stance toward herself and increase motivation toward therapeutic change.

The session includes a fair amount of review of diagnostic and treatment information; nonetheless we recommend maintaining a caring dialogue rather than a didactic listing of symptoms. Likewise, you have leeway about the specific examples or metaphors used in this session; the crucial feature for adherence is to provide specific and salient examples to aid the patient in developing a model for depression and the initial stage of the change process. If Session 1 is successful, the patient will be able to begin viewing her symptoms from the perspective of a disorder rather than personal weakness and will begin to identify targets for intervention.

Therapist Note

■ *To help with the memory dysfunction that often accompanies depression, Session 1 is frequently recorded for the patient. Discuss recording and the purpose of recording at the beginning of the session. You will ask the patient to listen to the tape once before the next session.* ■

Review of Confidentiality Policy and Patient's Previous Treatments

The session opens with a review of confidentiality and limits to confidentiality for information or charting in psychotherapy (as per your clinic or state policy). Follow this review with a discussion of the patient's previous psychosocial treatments. If the patient has not been in previous treatment, skip ahead to the next section.

If the patient has been in previous psychotherapy, initiate a brief discussion of the type of treatments received, including the style of the previous therapist(s) and the specific elements that were or were not helpful. The goal is to help provide a transition between past treatment efforts and the current treatment, not to review years of treatment. After your patient describes her previous therapy, we recommend that you summarize some of the salient points described by her, with attention to styles, habits, and strategies that the patient believes lead to depression, as well as styles or modalities of treatment that have been successful in the past. Ideally you will be able to compare and contrast stylistic aspects of past and current treatment. If the patient has been in previous insight-oriented treatment, discuss how this insight might be applied to therapy. For example, you might say something like the following:

> *One thing we will try to do is use some of this information to our advantage in your treatment, but the general style of treatment with me may be very different from what you have had in the past. In this treatment, I am going to try to be fairly active; that is, in certain sessions I may talk a lot. It is partly the goal of this treatment to teach you about common patterns in depression and how to shut down these patterns. This means that our therapy will involve more than talking; it will involve doing. Given that you have been frustrated by (element of previous treatment), you may especially like the focused approach we will try to follow in this treatment. In short, we will be discussing emotional, thought, and behavioral patterns that either serve you well or hurt you and your mood. Our goal is to increase the patterns that help you and decrease the patterns that hurt you through discussion and active practice.*

> *To make sure that we focus on patterns that currently get in your way, and to make sure that we have good continuity between sessions, we will start each treatment session by setting an agenda of things we want to work on. We will also keep close track of your mood, so we can tell when we are making progress and when we need to try harder.*

> *But I am getting a bit ahead of myself. Before we talk more about treatment, we should talk more about how we each see depression.*

Characterize depression as a syndrome that involves a common set of symptoms. Ensure that the patient can identify symptoms of depression as part of the larger syndrome. The acronym SIG E CAPS as described in Chapter 1 can be used to help you remember the range of symptoms you may want to review in addition to a sad or blue mood. You may also want to note associated symptoms such as irritability and anger and increased anxiety and worry.

Once the syndrome of depression has been discussed, the next goal is to help the patient develop an emotional symbol by which to identify the self-critical attitude that is common in depression. By having a clear notion of the style engendered by depression, the patient may be better able to react against this style. The example that follows uses the image of a stone gargoyle to typify depression. By suggesting that the gargoyle is whispering messages, you encourage the patient to attend to subtle, automatic thoughts. Of course, the strategy of personifying and differentially attending to various "voices" in one's head should be used only with patients who have intact reality testing; it is not an acceptable metaphor for patients who may be vulnerable to psychotic symptoms.

Although we encourage use of this metaphor, it is not a crucial feature of treatment. However, it is important to provide the patient with a clear characterization of the self-perpetuating aspects of depression, including a self-critical attitude.

Gargoyle Metaphor

I would like to tell you how I think about depression, because I see it in terms of a powerful image. I view it as a heavy, stone gargoyle, and if I am depressed, I can feel the weight of it on my shoulder, making everything I do harder. It makes it harder for me to be motivated, harder for me to get anything done, harder to get out of bed, and harder to concentrate. And one of the worst aspects of the gargoyle is that it isn't quiet. It is whispering in my ear. It is saying things like, "Look at you, you're depressed; what is the matter with you? You aren't

happy like other people." In particular, the depression gargoyle wants
you to blame yourself, to remind you of other times in your life when
things were going poorly, and to label everything that happens in
extreme terms. If something does not go well, the gargoyle says, "you
failed" or "you blew it" or "that was a disaster."

If you do something on track, the gargoyle will tell you that your
attempts are useless. If you feel bad, the gargoyle will tell you that this
is the way it will always be. If you make a mistake, the gargoyle will
tell you that this occurred because you are flawed. This is the gargoyle's
method. And remember, because you are depressed, many of the
messages whispered by the gargoyle will feel true. The gargoyle tries to
make everything appear darker, because if you blame yourself instead
of the depression gargoyle, it can just keep sitting on your shoulder,
weighing you down, and making everything harder.

Now that is how I view depression. How does this perspective, this
example of a depression gargoyle sound to you? Does it describe your
depression at all?

(Adapted from Otto, M. W. (2000) Stories and metaphors in cognitive-behavior therapy. *Cognitive and Behavioral Practice, 7,* 166–172.)

Discuss the metaphor with the patient, and if she can relate to it, continue with the following:

If you would like, we can then use this gargoyle image when we talk
about your depression. And in starting treatment for bipolar
depression, the trick is to make sure you do not buy into the gargoyle's
message. Over the next several weeks, I am going to ask you to listen
for the gargoyle's voice in the way you talk to yourself. And when you
hear this voice, I want you to label it as the voice of the "depression
gargoyle."

As an alternative to this voice, I am going to ask you to adopt the sort
of voice that I am using with you, a therapeutic voice. A voice that
assumes that you are currently hurting, coming for help, need to have
an ally, and need to treat yourself kindly while you are working at
change. You need encouragement and support as you change patterns
associated with depression. Don't let the gargoyle voice interfere with
this process.

A metaphor is only as useful as the way in which it strikes the patient, and serves as both a memory aid and an organizing image for applying therapy skills. This particular metaphor should not be used if you have any concern about a psychotic process in the patient or if you believe that the patient might overattend to the image. If the metaphor is used, you may want to specify that the gargoyle is "whispering" the negative thoughts. A whispered thought is consistent with the "automatic" way in which dysfunctional thoughts occur, and patients may need to stop and listen in on their thoughts to really notice their content. This stopping and listening in is consistent with the image of a gargoyle whispering. Also, when discussing the range of negative thoughts uttered by the gargoyle, you may want to include, *"The gargoyle may even be saying that therapy is a waste of time, that there is no use in wasting the doctor's time."* It is surprising how many patients will nod when their therapist introduces this thought. If so, you can be proud that you have identified a negative thought that may have been particularly hard for your patient to introduce into the session, and in voicing the thought and labeling it as the gargoyle's voice, you may have gone far to stop the patient from buying into this particular negative and potentially therapy-disrupting thought.

Depression About Depression

Discussions to externalize depression using the gargoyle metaphor provide a natural segue for discussing the phenomenon of "depression about depression." Discuss with the patient the tendency to become distraught, upset, and self-blaming about the experience of depression itself. Explain that getting angry at oneself for symptoms or becoming self-blaming has the potential of intensifying and lengthening the experience of depression (for research on this topic, see Dent & Teasdale, 1988).

Biased Thinking

Discuss that depression about depression is just one aspect of the general cognitive biases that occur with depression. Explain that depression generally brings with it negative views toward the self, more negative evaluations of situations, events, and the future, as well as more pessimistic memories of one's past. Provide a concrete example of the sort of memory biases that are found in depression. For example, you may want to illustrate this memory bias with a personal story such as the following:

> *Let me give you an example. If you give me a word like "train" when I am in a sad or blue mood, I might think of this time when I was young and I went to Durango, Colorado. In Durango, there is a station for a train that goes through some steep and beautiful mountain passes. But in this particular memory, I remember visiting the train station with a girlfriend, after we had driven for hours in a car having a terrible argument. It was one of those arguments that leaves a person feeling hopeless and bereft; wanting to fix it but not knowing how. That mood was all over me, and I remember standing in Durango, looking at the train station, and being unable to enjoy it. And that is the sort of memory that may come up when I'm feeling sad already.*

> *If I am in a happy mood, I am likely to recall a different memory. I actually have a different memory of a train, the same train, but the memory takes place on a different trip to the Durango area. I had hiked into the mountains for a couple of hours, down to a valley to fish in a stream. Once I got all the way down there it turns out that the train tracks went right by. So I'd hiked two hours, I'm standing there in my hiking gear, and I hear the train coming; an old train, stream engine, and it comes by and I'm waving to the people on the train, but otherwise standing in the middle of a wilderness. It was a really nice moment, and this might be the sort of memory that comes to mind if I am in a better mood and you ask me to recall a memory about a train.*

> *Now, as you can imagine, the way that I feel after having one or the other of these memories is very different: one leads me to happiness and memories of being outdoors and having fun, and the other reminds me of pain of a long-past relationship.*

Use your personal story to demonstrate how depression may feed on itself. When we are sad, it is easier to remember other sad events (the mood provides a link to other mood-similar memories). Once we have another sad memory, it makes it easier to continue to feel sad, or to feel like our mood has *always* been sad, or that life has *always* not gone well for us. Explain that these are natural reactions to moods. Emphasize, however, that it is important that we keep these mood effects on thoughts and memories in mind so that we can effectively undo depression.

The Role of Cognitions

Define cognitions as thoughts, images, and attitudes that occur on a moment-by-moment basis. Discuss that our perceptions and cognitions help define the world for us; that apart from the real world, our filtering and decisions about what is happening in the real world can greatly bias how we feel. Explain that cognitions do not have to be true to have a powerful effect on emotions. Give a relevant example, such as the following, also adapted from Otto, 2000:

> *Last night I had a tremendous meal. It was pasta with pesto sauce; delicious! Best of all, I didn't finish it. I have some home in my refrigerator now. The flavors have been melding over night. All I have to do is go home, heat it up, and I will have a tremendous dinner. I can see it, I can smell it, and I can almost taste it—the melding of the Parmesan, garlic, and basil. There is only one problem. I made up this story. I don't have pasta with pesto at home in the refrigerator. But this truth did not stop me, and perhaps you, from getting hungry for the pesto, and perhaps even salivating a little. And this is a good lesson about thoughts. They do not have to be true to have an effect on us. During treatment, I am going to have you keep this principle in mind: Thoughts can have effects on us and our emotions, even though they may not be true.*

Discuss with the patient that throughout therapy you are going to ask her to examine and monitor her mood. Explain that as part of treatment she will have to attend to and notice the types of cognitions that depression is helping her have. Together you will be judging thoughts not according to what feels true or feels false but rather you will discuss cognitions relative to their usefulness. Identify cognitions as another form of behavior (though special because this behavior occurs rapidly and in private). You may want to use the following dialogue to sum up:

> *Cognitions after all are our own thoughts, our own behavior. The whole point of our thinking about things is to help us in life, and right now, not only are a lot of your cognitions (because of the depression) not helping you but they are hurting you and your quality of life. So I'm going to ask you to start being appropriately selfish about your thoughts and to start guiding yourself with only those thoughts that help you, that are useful for you. In the upcoming treatment, we will give you very specific procedures to help this happen.*

Depression and Activity Levels

Talk about how depression can lead to a decrease in activity level. The feeling of not wanting to do things often keeps people away from positive events in their lives. For example, it is not uncommon for someone who is depressed to say, "I was going to do something, but I ended up just sitting in my room, staring at the wall for an hour and a half." Use the following dialogue in your discussion:

> *While you're staring at the wall, there are usually negative thoughts coursing through your head, and also there is the loss of what could have happened in that hour and a half. Generally, depression keeps you from getting out and potentially having good things happen in the world. Even if you do go out, those thought biases are often there to say to you, "You're not going to have fun anyway. What's the purpose? Why even bother?" Thoughts like these sap the fun of actually going out and make it more likely that during the first five minutes of being out you are looking around thinking, "I'm not having fun yet, what's the purpose?" Under these conditions, you can understand that it's really hard to have a positive event happen, either because you don't go out or because going out is so full of the negative thoughts that there's nothing there to re-spark pleasant feelings or pleasant memories.*

Explain that part of the management of depression is becoming aware of how depression insulates the patient from having positive experiences, as well the thoughts that prevent her from noticing that there are good things in her life or world.

Discuss that treatment will also focus on increasing activities. By applying cognitive strategies to life problems and examining activity levels, this program will help the patient achieve more enjoyment in her life.

Review CBT Model

In an open-ended fashion, discuss with the patient aspects of the CBT model that fit well with her experience of depression and those that do not. This discussion should lead fairly naturally to several targets for treatment during the first session (e.g., self-care).

Also, discuss other relevant targets (e.g., anxiety disorders) that will be part of the focus of treatment. Nonetheless, emphasize that the initial focus of intervention will be the major depression.

Self-Care

One target for intervention in the first session is negative cognitions about the self. The goal is to have the patient adopt a more forgiving attitude toward her symptoms as they occur. Remind her to use a therapeutic voice toward herself rather than listening to the "gargoyle."

In addition, pick one relevant example of how her thoughts may be serving her poorly, and discuss alternative thoughts that may prove more helpful to her when depressed. Inform the patient that she shares with you the direct role of therapist. Alternatively, to help the patient develop a better self-coaching perspective—following the assumption that people are often much less reasonable in the way they manage themselves relative to the way they manage others—you may want to place her in a role as head of a corporation who must figure out ways to give help to the people she employs. These employees—the patient in different roles—are unmotivated, and have difficulty concentrating, difficulty sleeping, and guilt. The role of the corporate CEO—the patient—is to help motivate and care for these employees. In short, you should strive to orient the patient toward self-care.

Self-Care around Suicidal Thoughts

Reiterate that self-care will be a central part of treatment, and discuss the role of suicidal thoughts as a symptom of depression. Protection against acting on these thoughts is a core feature of the therapeutic perspective. You are to help the patient link suicidal thoughts (if present) to the syndrome of depression and to discuss self-care within this context. Help the patient complete the Self-Care Worksheet for Suicidal Thoughts in the workbook, ensuring that she contracts for safety and agrees to use the suicide safety precautions outlined on the form.

Homework

✎ Have the patient complete the Weekly Activity Schedule found in the workbook as a first step toward understanding and modifying her usual activities.

✎ Have the patient review the Self-Care Worksheet for Suicidal Thoughts, if necessary.

✎ Have the patient listen to the session recording (if completed) at least once before the next session.

Closing the Session

Discuss with the patient any questions that she may have about the session, and invite her to identify any aspects of the model that do not seem to fit with her expectations. Also ask her to identify any aspects of the homework that seem especially hard. Remind the patient that the purpose is not to do "perfectly well" on the assignments. The assignments may be somewhat difficult; however, the purpose is to attempt the assignments and discuss difficulties as well as successes.

Chapter 4

Session 2: Mood Charting and Activity Scheduling

(Corresponds to chapter 2 of the workbook)

Materials Needed

- Mood Chart

- Pleasant Events List

Outline

- Introduce agenda setting and set agenda

- Review patient's symptoms and Self-Care Worksheet for Suicidal Thoughts

- Present the Mood Chart

- Discuss activity monitoring and Pleasant Events List

- Present the coaching story

- Summarize session

- Assign homework

Therapist Note

■ *For this and all following sessions, consider whether a recording of the session will serve the patient well (to aid consolidation of each week's session by having the patient listen to the session during the week).* ■

When working with bipolar patients, maintaining structure in the session is sometimes a challenging task. Setting an agenda early in the session, structures the time in session and also ensures that topics included in the treatment protocol are covered. A collaborative approach works best when setting an agenda. Although certain topics are required by the protocol at each session, there is some flexibility in addressing specific problem areas. It is important to explain to patients the rationale for agenda setting and to engage them in the process of setting the agenda.

In order to set an agenda, therapist's need to be updated on the current status of the patient, including reactions to last week's home practices, if assigned. Accordingly, early session topics should include a "mood check." This is best done by reviewing the patient's Mood Chart. The Mood Chart is a recommended part of this program; formal introduction to charting in the context of CBT occurs later in this session. Mood charting provides a systematic assessment of daily changes in mood, sleep patterns, and medication compliance, as well as a report on daily stressors. Ideally, by viewing the patient's Mood Chart, you will get a rapid snapshot of the past week. In this way, you can quickly get a sense of problem areas and add them to the agenda for discussion. Many patients also find that presenting the Mood Chart to their therapist saves time in the session for issues of greatest importance to them. Rather than a lengthy dialogue recapping mood changes and weekly events, the mood chart allows a quick transition to specific topics. Of course, this strategy is helpful only if the patient complies with completion of the Mood Chart. (See Chapter 2 for more information on dealing with compliance issues). Including a review of the Mood Chart at the beginning of each session tends to improve compliance.

Review of previous homework also informs each session's agenda, and compliance for homework improves if the patient expects that it will be checked at each session. A brief review of previous homework also builds a bridge from the previous session's material, providing a sense of continuity between sessions. This is particularly important for bipolar patients who may be easily distracted or have difficulty recalling previous session's material. As an aside, many techniques can be used to assist the patient in remembering session material, such as having him listen to audiotapes of sessions or record notes from each session in the space provided in the workbook.

The following vignette illustrates one way of introducing agenda setting:

Case Vignette

T: Near the beginning of each session, we will be setting an agenda, deciding together what topics we will discuss. This helps us make sure that we will cover the areas of most importance each week. At each session, there will be certain topics that I will want to discuss with you. But, of course, this is your therapy, and I would like you to let me know about specific problem areas that you would like to address. In other words, you and I will work together to come up with a plan for each session. Sounds okay with you so far?

P: Yeah.

T: Okay, prior to setting each session's agenda, we will start by covering some routine things. I will be asking you about your mood, and checking to see if you had any difficulties with your sleep and medications. Today, I will be showing you a way to keep track of this on a daily basis, using a form called a Mood Chart. So, at the beginning of each session's agenda, I will check in with you to see how you have been feeling over the past week, and I will ask to see your Mood Chart.

P: OK.

T: This is a very active treatment, so at each session we will be discussing ways to follow up on what we have covered through the use of home practice assignments. At the beginning of each session, we will briefly discuss the previous week's session and review your home practice. So, let's go ahead and talk about setting our agenda for today.

Discuss today's agenda and explain that this session will be devoted to reviewing the patient's symptoms and expanding on some of the concepts introduced last session, in particular the role of thoughts in depression and other negative mood states. Naturally, the agenda should include topics and concerns expressed by the patient. The concept of the agenda should be presented as an endeavor shared by both the therapist and the patient.

Review of Patient's Symptoms and Self-Care Worksheet for Suicidal Thoughts

Reviewing symptoms includes a discussion of the patient's attitude toward his symptoms, with attention to the presence of depression about depression. In particular, you should examine whether the patient:

- understands his symptoms in the context of a depression syndrome

- is responding to symptoms with self-depreciation or self-blame

- made any progress in adopting a more therapeutic attitude toward symptoms during the previous week

- was able to use the "gargoyle" (or similar model) in examining his self-talk around symptoms

In addition, discuss whether the patient has any modifications to the Self-Care Worksheet for Suicidal Thoughts (when this form is finalized, both you and the patient should retain a copy). In discussing these items, you should further model the attitude of therapeutic problem solving.

Mood Chart

Introduce the concept of a Mood Chart. Completion of a Mood Chart provides both you and the patient with a means of tracking his mood patterns and everyday life events that may be impacting his mood state. The Mood Chart is a tool that the patient can use to report his symptoms in a more efficient manner to care providers. It also serves as an effective tool for predicting the future course of bipolar illness and warning signs associated with mood changes. The Mood Chart should be reviewed at the beginning of each session. A blank copy is provided for the patient in the corresponding workbook.

The following vignette illustrates the presenting of the Mood Chart to a patient and strategies to enhance compliance with daily completion.

Case Vignette

T: Do you recall during our last session that I asked many questions about your mood and fluctuations from depression to elevation?

P: Yes, the questions were overwhelming. I really couldn't give you much information because my mood changes all the time and it has been that way for years. There is no way for me to keep track of it!

T: I agree. It can be quite difficult to recall your mood and its fluctuations. I am bringing this up again because I would like to share with you a way to track your mood and mood changes more closely. I am recommending you use something called a Mood Chart. (Refer patient to the blank Mood Chart in Chapter 2 of the workbook.)

P: This looks very complicated to complete. I am not going to have the time to do this.

T: It may look complicated and time consuming, but it can take as little as 30 seconds a day to complete. I realize that there are a lot of boxes and blanks, but this one chart is for a whole month. You actually only need to complete one row per day. Let's go over how you might do that.

Review the instructions in the workbook, and go over each column of the Mood Chart. You may want to suggest that the patient set up some prompts to remind himself to complete the chart every morning and night. For example, he can leave reminder notes somewhere he is bound to see them (e.g. bathroom mirror, refrigerator, or front door). It might be helpful to use several prompts at first.

The patient may also forget to bring the Mood Chart to sessions. Hopefully, reviewing the Mood Chart at the start of every session will underscore its significance in treatment. In addition, you can help the patient set up prompts at home to enhance memory for bringing the Mood Chart, and therefore his workbook to session (e.g., leaving himself a note, putting the workbook somewhere he'll see it). Again, the patient may want to "overdo it" with the prompts until he is in the habit of using and bringing the chart and workbook.

Stress to the patient the importance of bringing the Mood Chart with him to every visit. Remind him that the chart serves as a great summary of the questions that his care providers will be asking him. Instead of asking him those same questions over and over in every session, you can just refer to the Mood Chart and ask questions from there.

The patient might be overwhelmed by the perceived complexity of completing the Mood Chart. Reassure the patient that it can take as little as 30 seconds a day to complete, and have him practice in session to underscore this point (a sample Mood Chart in the workbook provides guidance). Moreover, the patient may become confused about making two separate mood ratings (one for the highest point of the day and one for the lowest point of the day). To lessen confusion, review completion of this section several times in session.

Activity Monitoring and Pleasant Events List

Discuss with the patient his level of activity during the monitoring period. If the patient forgot his homework, spend session time to complete an average weekday and average weekend day of activities on the Weekly Activity Schedule. Discuss the patient's thoughts about the observed activity level (overactivity or underactivity, deficits of pleasurable events, etc.) and its impact on mood. Ask the patient to think about some of the enjoyable activities that he used to do or would like to start doing.

Begin to discuss the impact of buffering events and pleasant activities on mood. Explain that buffering events are those small activities that a person does week to week that can reliably break up the stress of the week. These activities can be almost anything—watching a favorite television show, taking time to read, working on a hobby, spending time with a friend, scheduling a regular night to go out to dinner—anything that can happen with some regularity. Some people pick a time of the day or a time of the week for such an activity and then change the activity each week, depending on their interests.

This session's homework will include a review of the Pleasant Events List. You may use the following sample dialogue to present this list to the patient:

In the next few sessions, we will start building in more of these buffering activities. I want you to start thinking about some pleasurable events that you may want to add to your life. This is important for treating depression because depression has a way of sapping motivation and sucking away pleasurable activities in a person's life. In your workbook, you will find a list of pleasant events. As part of your home practice, I would like you to review this list for things you haven't done for a while or would like to do. This does not mean you have to have motivation for these things right now—after all, you are depressed—but I'd like to find out about some of the things you might enjoy as you start feeling better. As you see here, this form has listed a number of activities that people sometimes enjoy, and some space at the end to write in additional activities.

Have the patient go through the Pleasant Events List and circle any activities he thinks he might enjoy, making darker circles around the items he think he might enjoy the most. Discuss why and why not the items look interesting.

Coaching Story

The last intervention in Session 2 is the coaching story (adapted from Otto, 2000). This story provides initial training in the evaluation of thoughts and the substitution of more adaptive self-talk. Once established, the coaching story serves as a useful metaphor for discussing cognitive restructuring. In particular, the coaching story serves as a useful guide for the tone and content of effective self-talk, and cognitive restructuring interventions can be introduced or discussed in terms of *"how did you coach yourself this week?"*

Story telling is aided by the effective use of changes in vocal tone and tempo, as well as theatrical pauses and gestures. The goal is to make the story compelling and memorable, so that the patient can apply its message over the following weeks.

This is a story about little league baseball. I talk about little league baseball because of the amazing parents and coaches involved. And by "amazing" I don't mean good. I mean extreme.

But this story doesn't start with the coaches or the parents; it starts with Johnny, who is a little league player in the outfield. His job is to catch fly balls and return them to the infield players. On the day of our story, Johnny is in the outfield and "crack!"—one of the players on the other team hits a fly ball. The ball is coming to Johnny. Johnny raises his glove. The ball is coming to him, coming to him . . . and it goes over his head. Johnny misses the ball, and the other team scores a run.

Now there are a number of ways a coach can respond to this situation. Let's take Coach A first. Coach A is the type of coach who will come out on the field and shout: "I can't believe you missed that ball! Anyone could have caught it! My dog could have caught it! You screw up like that again and you'll be sitting on the bench! That was lousy!" Coach A then storms off the field.

At this point, Johnny is standing in the outfield and, if he is at all similar to me, he is tense, tight, trying not to cry, and praying that another ball is not hit to him. If a ball does come to him, Johnny will probably miss it. After all, he is tense, tight, and may see four balls coming at him because of the tears in his eyes. If we are Johnny's parents, we may see more profound changes after the game. Johnny, who typically places his baseball glove on the mantel, now throws it under his bed. And before the next game, he may complain that his stomach hurts, that perhaps he should not go to the game. This is the scenario with Coach A.

Now let's go back to the original event and play it differently. Johnny has just missed the ball, and now Coach B comes out on the field. Coach B says: "Well, you missed that one. Here is what I want you to remember: high balls look like they are farther away than they really are. Also, it is much easier to run forward than to back-up. Because of this, I want you to prepare for the ball by taking a few extra steps backwards. As the ball gets closer you can step into it if you need to. Also, try to catch it at chest level, so you can adjust your hand if you misjudge the ball. Let's see how you do next time." Coach B then leaves the field.

How does Johnny feel? Well, he is not happy. After all, he missed the ball—but there are a number of important differences from the way he felt with Coach A. He is not as tense or tight, and if a fly ball does come to him, he knows what to do differently to catch it. And because he does not have tears in his eyes, he may actually see the ball and catch it.

So, if we were the type of parent who wanted Johnny to make the Major Leagues, we would pick Coach B because he teaches Johnny how to be a more effective player. Johnny knows what to do differently, may catch more balls, and may excel in the game.

But if we didn't care whether Johnny made the Major Leagues— because baseball is a game, and one is supposed to be able to enjoy a game—then we would again pick Coach B. We would pick Coach B because we care whether Johnny enjoys the game. With Coach B, Johnny knows what to do differently; he is not tight, tense, and ready to cry; he may catch a few balls; and he may enjoy the game. He may also continue to place his glove on the mantel.

Now, while we may all select Coach B for Johnny, we rarely choose the voice of Coach B for the way we talk to ourselves. Think about your last mistake. Did you say, "I can't believe I did that! I am so stupid! What a jerk!"? These are "Coach A" thoughts, and they have many of the same effects on us as Coach A has on Johnny. These thoughts make us feel tense and tight, may make us feel like crying, and rarely help us do better in the future. Remember, even if you were only concerned about productivity (making the Major Leagues), you would still pick Coach B. And if you were concerned with enjoying life, with guiding yourself effectively for both joy and productivity, you certainly would pick Coach B.

During the next week, I would like you to listen to see how you are coaching yourself. If you hear Coach A, remember this story and see if you can replace "Coach A" thoughts with "Coach B" thoughts.

The strategy of closing the session with the coaching story is designed to make the story the most salient feature of the session. The goal is to maximize the patient's memory cues for the story so that cognitive restructuring during the week will naturally occur in relation to the message.

Session Summary

At the conclusion of each session, present the patient with a brief summary of the topics covered and review important points. In the early stages of treatment, it is usually the therapist who provides this summary. However, in later stages, it is more helpful to ask the patient for a brief summary of what he will take away from the session.

Take a few minutes to review with the patient the most salient points of today's session. It is helpful to consolidate the information and make sure that the patient understands and remembers the important points.

Homework

✎ Ask patient to review the Pleasant Events List and continue to monitor his activities using the Weekly Activity Schedule in the workbook.

✎ Ask patient to pay attention to the way he coaches himself and to replace any "Coach A" thoughts he may have with "Coach B" thoughts instead.

✎ Assign listening to the audiotape of the session (if completed).

Chapter 5 | *Session 3: Cognitive Restructuring—Part I*

(Corresponds to chapter 3 of the workbook)

Materials Needed

- List of cognitive errors
- Pleasant Events List
- Weekly Activity Schedule
- Thought Record

Outline

- Set agenda
- Review Mood Chart
- Review patient's progress
- Review homework
- Review Pleasant Events List and introduce activity scheduling
- Discuss the list of cognitive errors
- Introduce self-monitoring and the Thought Record
- Summarize session
- Assign homework

Set Agenda

Open the session with information on the general topics to be covered, incorporating the patient's agenda items with those in this manual. (See Session 2 for more instructions on agenda setting.) You may use the following dialogue to set this session's agenda:

Well, as we will always try to do, I want to start the session by reviewing your Mood Chart, checking in on your reactions to last week's session, and then seeing what topics you have for the agenda. Does anything stand out for you that is important for us to cover?

For my part, I would like to review your reactions to the coaching story and to talk about some other strategies I would like you to have for evaluating and changing how you approach your thinking habits. Remember that in this therapy, I am going to pay extra attention to how you are viewing the world and yourself because of the dramatic effects depression can have on thinking style.

I also want to spend some time talking more about your weekly schedule and to see what we can do to try to give you increased moments of pleasure. Does this sound like a good plan?

Mood Chart Review

Review symptom levels since the previous session using the patient's Mood Chart. Discuss with the patient her attitudes toward symptoms, evaluating the presence of dysfunctional cognitions about moods. Discuss any episodes of medication noncompliance using the medication noncompliance protocol (see Chapter 2).

Progress Review

Initiate a review of the patient's progress with a discussion of the use of the coaching story. For example, you may say:

Last week, I presented you with a story about coaching styles. Tell me what you thought of the story and what you noticed about your own style of self-talk during the past week. Did you tend to talk to yourself like Coach A or Coach B?

Ask the patient about her experience with the different coaching styles. The goal of this discussion is to elicit from the patient her application of the coaching story, with specific encouragement of adoption of a Coach B style. If necessary, reiterate relevant parts from the story.

Homework Review

Review the patient's Weekly Activity Schedule from last week, as well as the activities she circled on the Pleasant Events List. The goal of this review is to identify a number of activities the patient may wish to introduce or reintroduce into her life.

Emphasize to the patient that treatment involves trying to increase her pleasure in life. Ask the patient to select one pleasant event to introduce into her life in the next week and select target days when this event may be added. Ask the patient to pay attention to how it feels to complete the activity or event, instructing her to pay extra attention to any pleasure that may be achieved, no matter how small. Acknowledge to the patient that pleasure may be diminished by the depression, but that it is nonetheless important to begin to reintroduce a focus on pleasure.

Identifying Cognitive Errors

Introduce the Burns' list of cognitive errors as examples of typical cognitive styles that support depressogenic thinking patterns. A copy of this list is included here, as well as in the patient workbook. The goal of introducing the list is to illustrate ways in which one's thinking style may be skewed in a negative way. The goal is not to have the patient dogmatically learn to classify a thought as certain type of error (e.g., All-or-nothing thinking, Overgeneralization) but to increase her awareness and ability to recognize these types of thoughts in general. This is a first step in helping the patient identify the connections between thoughts, feelings, and behaviors.

The Burns' list provides you as the therapist with a means to convey that people, not just the patient, make cognitive errors. The list also helps to provide the patient with the initial "sound" and "feel" of dysfunctional thoughts so that she can better identify these cognitions when they occur. The labeling of the different styles of cognitive errors provides the patient with guidance for honing self-monitoring. With a better classification system, patients may be more able to identify cognitive errors when they occur, "Oh, this sounds kind of like that example where..." You should take time to exemplify the types of errors that people make in their thinking and self-evaluation, but without pressing for dogmatic learning of the types of errors.

The following are adapted from *Feeling Good: The New Mood Therapy* (Burns, 1999).

All-or-Nothing Thinking (Black-and-White Thinking)

You think in black and white terms; there are no gray areas. This type of thinking is unrealistic because things are seldom all or nothing, good or bad.

Overgeneralization

You assume that a one-time negative occurrence will happen again and again. You use words like "always" or "never" to make generalizations.

Mental Filter

You focus exclusively on negative details and ignore anything positive. Since you are filtering out the positives, you see the entire situation as negative.

Disqualifying the Positive

You turn positives into negatives by insisting they "don't count." This allows you to maintain your negative outlook despite positive experiences.

Jumping to Conclusions

In the absence of solid evidence, you jump to a negative conclusion. There are two types of this: "mind reading" and the "fortune teller error."

Mind Reading

You assume that you know what someone else is thinking. You are so convinced that the person is having a negative reaction to you, you don't even take the time to confirm your guess.

The Fortune Teller Error

You act as a fortune teller who only predicts the worst for you. You then treat your unrealistic prediction as if it were a proven fact.

Magnification (Catastrophizing) or Minimization

You magnify negative things, blowing their importance out of proportion. The outcome of an event appears catastrophic to you.

You minimize positive things, shrinking down their significance. You make good experiences out to be smaller than they are.

Emotional Reasoning

You take your emotions as proof of the way things really are. You assume something is true because you feel it is.

"Should" Statements

You build your expectations with "shoulds," "musts," and "oughts." When you don't follow through, you feel guilty. When others disappoint you, you feel angry and resentful.

Labeling and Mislabeling

You label yourself or someone else, rather than just identifying the behavior.

You mislabel an event by using inaccurate and emotionally extreme language.

Personalization

You take responsibility for things that you don't have control over. You feel guilty because you assume a negative event is your fault.

Case Vignette

See the following case vignette for an illustration of how to facilitate discussion about cognitive errors.

T: This is a list of some common distortions people make in their thinking when depressed. We are going to briefly review these types of thinking errors in order to give you some examples of the way in which depression may be influencing your thinking. OK?

P: OK

T: One type of cognitive error is All-or-Nothing Thinking. This type of error, also known as Black-and-White thinking, refers to seeing things as either completely good or completely bad, with no gray or middle ground. An example of this would involve a person viewing herself as either a complete success or a complete failure. Unfortunately, life is often not so clear-cut and very few individuals succeed or fail at absolutely everything. Most of life is in shades of gray. Can you think of any examples of how you might think in black-and-white terms?

P: No. Not really.

T: Well, how about earlier in today's session when you were saying that your life is worthless now that you have bipolar disorder.

P: It does seem like everything is screwed up now.

T: There, you have said it well for discussing black-and-white thinking. You said, "EVERYTHING is screwed up now." Can you think of any examples of things that may still be working ok?

P: Well, my attention is on the things the bipolar disorder is affecting, but I guess my life isn't completely changed.

T: Let's look at what things may still be working.

P: Well, I guess I am still a good parent and my kids seem to care about me. I am changing jobs, but it seems like employers are still interested in me.

T: Great. You just changed your extreme thinking to a more balanced view. With just a moment's thinking, you realized that saying "EVERYTHING is screwed up" is not accurate. I want you to remember this example as one way your thoughts may not be accurate. Instead of presenting a balanced view of your own circumstances, it may be easy, particularly when depressed, to overfocus on just a few of the facts. If you had to restate your unbalanced version of your life ("EVERYTHING is screwed up") in a more accurate fashion, what would you say?

P: Well, some things are screwed up, but some things do seem to be working.

T: That's it. The importance of catching all-or-nothing thinking is that it is much easier to live in a world where some things are screwed up and some things are working, than to try to cope with a worldview that EVERYTHING is screwed up.

P: Yeah, it doesn't sound so bad.

Self-Monitoring and the Thought Record

Self-monitoring of cognitions is a central strategy for providing patients with a structure for completing cognitive restructuring. The Thought Record provides a tangible reminder of self-monitoring assignments and the step-by-step approach to be adopted in examining thoughts. In addition, the Thought Record helps ensure that patients will have the opportunity to examine their thoughts in the more objective context of a written assignment. You may use either of the following sample dialogues to underscore the difference between thinking about cognitive restructuring and writing out the assignment.

> *As you well know, if thinking about something were the same as writing it, many of us would be famed novelists. But writing is different than just thinking about something. Writing slows down your thought process and gives you a product (the written sentences) that you can then read back to yourself and consider in a way that is different from just turning over a thought in your head. So, to help you adopt a very objective perspective on your thoughts, I am going to emphasize the importance of writing out this assignment, not just thinking about it, so that you can clearly evaluate some of the automatic thoughts we have been talking about.*

> *The cognitive restructuring practice that I am going to ask you to complete requires you to write out your thoughts. Now, writing out a thought has value all on its own. I like to think about some negative thoughts similar to the way I think about certain monster movies. In many monster movies, the monster is always more powerful and frightening in the dark. Think of Dracula. Dracula is very frightening and dangerous in the dark, but if you get him out in the light of day, he turns to dust. Negative thoughts are like this. They have more power when they can just flit through our minds. By writing down your thoughts, you will have the chance to examine them out of your head, in the bright light of the page where you wrote them. I think this will make it easier to view your thoughts objectively, to decide whether your thoughts are accurate or whether they are leading your emotions astray.*

Over the next several sessions, you will teach the patient to use the Thought Record to monitor, evaluate, and modify her thoughts, with the goal of improving her mood. The record consists of multiple columns used to separately document (a) thought content, (b) the feelings associated with these thoughts, (c) the evaluation of the accuracy of thoughts, and (d) more accurate alternative thoughts. Review of Thought Records in session also forms the basis of active, cognitive restructuring rehearsal, which is a core feature of the first phase of treatment. In all cases, it is important to complete cognitive restructuring using specific situations and examples. The following case vignette is an example of how to introduce the Thought Record and rehearse cognitive restructuring.

Case Vignette

T: The Thought Record will help you identify your negative thoughts, how you feel when you think these particular thoughts, how to evaluate them to see just how accurate they are, and then how to generate alternative thoughts.

P: That sounds like a tall order. I don't know what I am thinking half of the time.

T: It sounds like a lot to learn, but I will show you how to use the Thought Record in a step-by-step fashion. We will focus first on identifying your dysfunctional thoughts and your associated feelings. Only later will we focus on evaluating the accuracy of your thoughts and begin generating alternative ways of viewing events. Let's use an example to get you started. Do you remember when you came into session today and said you have been sad and frustrated since you spoke with your mom on the phone this morning?

P: Yes, I really have been. It seems like I always get upset when I talk to my mom.

T: Well, I would like you to try to think back to this morning and your phone conversation with her. Try to remember the point when you started to feel sad. Can you do that?

P: The conversation started and things went pretty well. Then she started asking me about my job search. She just doesn't seem to get it. I am doing the best I can to find a job.

T: Okay. When she asked you about the job search, do you recall what went through your mind or what you were thinking about?

P: I really don't know. But every time she asks me about my job situation it always upsets me.

T: That is a good observation. When we experience a change in mood or an intense emotion, we are often engaging in automatic thoughts that we are not likely aware of. So when your mom was asking you about the job search, you know it made you upset. Right?

P: Yes.

If the patient has difficulty reporting thoughts, paradoxical questioning can be used to help elicit thoughts. For example, in the following statement, the therapist suggests a thought that is likely to be opposite to what the patient was actually thinking in the situation with her mother.

T: So I bet you were having some thoughts when you began to feel upset or what you also called sad and frustrated. Maybe you were thinking about how proud your mom is that you are working so hard to find a job!

P: Yeah right! She is not supportive at all. Actually, when she asked me about my job search, I was thinking that I will never find a job and that I am going to have to depend on my parents forever.

T: So you thought about your parents having to support you, what else?

P: Then I thought about what a loser I am because I don't have a job yet. And how successful all my friends are and how happy they are at their jobs. I thought about how pathetic my life is.

T: Well, there you go. You came up with what you were thinking when you started to feel sad and frustrated. As I said before, when you notice a shift in your feelings, you may be engaging in automatic thoughts that are not useful. Take notice and describe the feelings to yourself and label them if possible. A helpful question to ask yourself is, "What is going through my mind right now?" Let's see if you can transfer this example onto the Thought Record.

P: So where do I write this?

T: I like to start with the second column, the feelings. First put down your feelings of sadness and frustration.

P: OK.

T: Now write out the thoughts that you told me. You said that you were having thoughts like, "I am a loser" and "My life is pathetic." What do you think of those thoughts now that you have them down in black and white?

P: Wow, they look pretty severe.

T: That is part of the value of writing out thoughts. It gives you a chance to see just how nasty you may talk to yourself at times. How do you think most people would feel when faced by thoughts of this kind?

P: I would imagine they would feel like hell, but what is the alternative? Do you want me to go around all of the time thinking, "Oh my life is so good?" I really wonder sometimes whether I will have a good life or whether I am a loser.

T: Let's take a moment and consider that question. You are in a position right now where you are rather freely using the term "loser" to describe yourself, apparently because you haven't yet found a job. If you are going to use a term like that, you had better define it for me. What is a loser?

P: I don't know. I guess a loser is a person, you know, who never does anything worthwhile, never achieves anything.

T: And how true is that for you, that you never do anything worthwhile?

P: Well, I don't have a job.

T: That wasn't what I asked. I know you don't have a job right now, but is it true that you never do anything worthwhile?

P: (laughing) No. I actually do a number of things right, and to tell the truth I got one job offer, it was just that the job was lousy.

T: OK, so you are telling me that, according to your definition, you do not meet the criteria for a loser?

P: Right, but sometimes I feel like a loser.

T: Ahhh, that is an important distinction. You know logically that you are not a loser, but at times you FEEL like a loser.

P: Yeah.

T: And can you think of any reasons why your FEELINGS about yourself may be especially negative.

P: So you think this is part of the depression.

T: Yes, I do think that you are primed right now to FEEL like lots of things are not going well. That is part of depression. And, because you are depressed, I want to be especially careful about buying into these feelings and coaching yourself with words like LOSER.

P: It can't be good for my depression, can it?

T: No, it can't. Thinking about it now, what might be a more accurate way of coaching yourself around not having a job?

P: Well, I might say, this feels like hell, but I did get one offer. But isn't this just thinking "happy thoughts"?

T: No, it is more like thinking accurate thoughts. Thinking happy thoughts would be more like, "It is a bright cheery day, and I will get a job today for sure."

P: (laughs)

T: I am not trying to get you to think happy thoughts; instead, I am trying to help your thoughts serve you by being accurate. I want your thoughts to be useful for you, and I know calling yourself a loser just does not help, especially when you are depressed. Remember, it is important that you act as a therapist for yourself, to guide yourself with your thoughts.

P: To be a better "Coach B."

T: Exactly. And now that you had a chance to evaluate your thoughts, what is your mood when you think about not having a job.

P: Well, it isn't good, but at least I don't feel like dirt.

T: This is a good start. Now let's talk about how you can apply what we talked about in home practice.

Figure 5.1 shows what the Thought Record for the patient in the preceding case example would look like.

Situation	Emotion	Automatic thought	Evaluation of automatic thought	Re-rate emotion
(Describe the event that led to the unpleasant emotion)	(Specify sad, angry, etc., and rate the emotion from 0% to 100%)	(Write the automatic thought and rate your belief in the thought from 0% to 100%)	(Evaluate the accuracy of the automatic thought)	(Re-rate the emotion and your belief in the thought from 0% to 100%)
Spoke to my mom on the phone. She asked me about my job search.	Sad 90% Frustrated 95%	"I will never find a job and will have to rely on my parents forever." "I am a loser" Belief in thoughts = 95%	I actually did get one job offer, but it wasn't right for me. Even though I may feel like a loser, I have experienced success in my life.	Sad 25% Frustrated 40%

Figure 5.1

Example of Completed Thought Record

Eliciting Automatic Thoughts

When patients have initial difficulty identifying automatic thoughts, it is often helpful to "bring the situation into the session" by completing a brief role-play or, as in the preceding example, to imagine that the situation is occurring at the moment. For this imagination exercise, use the present tense, and take time to elicit the full range of thoughts before proceeding to a further step in cognitive restructuring. In general, you will be asking, *"What else are you thinking?"* or *"What other thoughts occur to you now that you thought of that?"* The goal is to get a full accounting of the thoughts in the moment, and when unclear, the affective meaning of the thoughts.

Session Summary

Take a few minutes to review with the patient the most salient points of today's session. It is helpful to consolidate the information and make sure that the patient understands and remembers the important points.

Homework

✎ Instruct patient to review the list of cognitive errors in the workbook.

✎ Have patient use the Thought Record to monitor her thoughts over the course of the next week. For now, the patient should only fill out the first three columns of the record (situation, emotion, and automatic thought only).

✎ Have patient continue monitoring her activities and recording them on the Weekly Activity Schedule in the workbook.

Chapter 6 — Session 4: Cognitive Restructuring—Part II

(Corresponds to chapter 4 of the workbook)

Materials Needed

- Thought Record
- Pleasant Events List
- Weekly Activity Schedule

Outline

- Set agenda
- Review Mood Chart
- Review homework
- Discuss evaluation or challenge of cognitive errors or negative thinking
- Discuss activity planning
- Summarize session
- Assign homework

Set Agenda

Open the session with review of the patient's Mood Chart and response to homework, combined with information on the general topics to be covered, incorporating the patient's agenda items with those in this manual. (See Session 2 for more instructions on agenda setting.)

Mood Chart Review

Review symptom levels since the previous session using the patient's Mood Chart. Discuss with the patient his attitudes toward symptoms, evaluating the presence of dysfunctional cognitions about moods. Discuss any episodes of medication noncompliance using the medication noncompliance protocol (see Chapter 2).

Homework Review

Homework review should begin with a reminder of what was discussed in the last session. For example:

> *Last week, we discussed how to identify your thoughts and provided some examples of cognitive errors. We agreed you would keep track of your cognitions using the Thought Record. How did your monitoring of thoughts go over the past week?*

Follow-up questions should focus on any difficulties in identifying thoughts and whether Burns' classification system offered any guidance. A discussion and review of thought monitoring can be followed by a similar discussion on activity monitoring.

If the patient was able to complete the pleasant activity scheduled during the previous session, discuss how it went. If not, problem solve around obstacles to completion. Review the patient's other activities and assess cognitions surrounding these events.

Evaluating or Challenging Thoughts

Introduce evaluation of thoughts as the next step in cognitive restructuring. Explain that once the patient is able to identify thoughts that are related to feelings of depression, then the accuracy of these thoughts is to be questioned. Review the thoughts recorded on the patient's

Thought Record and look for common themes. Allow the patient to respond and elaborate on these. Discuss strategies for challenging thoughts including asking the following questions:

- *"What evidence do you have that this thought is true?"*

- *"What evidence do you have against this thought?"*

Encourage in-session practice using the same line of questioning for other automatic thoughts that were documented in the previous week's homework. Use the next column in the Thought Record to write down evidence for and against each thought. Assist the patient with a few examples and then allow him to complete several independently. The following case vignette illustrates the process of weighing the evidence:

Case Vignette

T: On several occasions over the past week, you listed a particular automatic thought about your girlfriend not caring about you and using you until someone better comes along.

P: Yeah. It has been that way for awhile now. I am sure she is out looking for someone better, which probably won't be too hard to find. She doesn't really care about me.

T: Here on the Thought Record you wrote that you felt that way last night. What evidence is there that the thought that your girlfriend doesn't care about you is true?

P: Well, she said she was going to call me at 9:00 and she didn't. She knew I was having a really hard day and she still didn't call when she said she would. She didn't care if I was okay or not.

T: Okay. Let's consider another angle here for a minute. What evidence do you have that your girlfriend does care about you?

P: I already told you she doesn't.

T: I know you feel that way, and you've told me some things she does that might suggest that, but try hard to come up with something even if you aren't sure if they are signs that she cares. What kind of things does she say or do that suggests she might care about you?

P: Well . . . she compliments me a lot. She is also pretty supportive. She even took me out to dinner last weekend to celebrate my completing another semester at school.

T: So, based on what you just told me, there are times when she doesn't follow through with a commitment, like calling you. Yet, there are other times when she makes an effort to remember special occasions. Is this correct?

P: Well yeah.

T: It sounds like you have evidence both for and against the automatic thought that your girlfriend does not care for you.

P: Yeah, it felt true, but I really didn't think then of any examples of times when she treated me better.

Alternative Strategies for Evaluating Thoughts

A range of strategies are available for helping patients evaluate their thoughts. At times, evaluation can be aided by logical inquiry, asking the patient to evaluate the thought relative to some external criteria (e.g., clarification of the definition of a "loser" so that the patient can compare the label to a fuller set of criteria).

Alternatively, you may want to guide the patient toward thought evaluation by simply providing an emotional context for questioning the thought. For example, you may exclaim, *"Wow that is one nasty label."* Or *"Ouch, what do you think of that thought?"* The exclamation provides the patient with a salient cue that there was something painful about the thought and that something that painful deserves scrutiny.

A third method may be to link the thought back to a useful metaphor. For instance, the concept of the gargoyle (Session 1) or Coach A (Session 2) can be used as a strategy to help the patient stop and examine the thought, its accuracy, and its effect on mood.

The patient may also have difficulty being objective enough to generate evidence for and against some thoughts. In this case, encourage the patient to distance himself from the situation, asking him to approach it as if he was offering advice to a friend as in the following case vignette.

Case Vignette

T: If your friend was in your situation, if he failed his chemistry exam and thought that he ought to drop out of school because he wasn't "smart enough" to be in college, what would you say to him?

P: I really don't know.

T: Would you say "Yeah I agree that failing one test suggests that you are not smart enough to be here. You should drop out!"

P: No. I wouldn't do that! I would probably say "Come on, what about the 'B' that you got on the first exam? You helped tutor all of us for that one." Or, I may remind him that he had a pretty good GPA last semester and that he is getting at least a "B" in biology.

T: Do these same words apply to you?

P: Yeah, I guess they do.

T: So, if you are having trouble challenging your automatic thoughts, try thinking of what you would tell a friend. This strategy can help you to gain some objectivity in the situation.

Generating Ideas for Activity Planning

Review the Pleasant Events List and the patient's completed Weekly Activity Schedule as an aid for generating ideas for activity planning. The goal of activity planning is to increase the patient's interaction with his environment through a well-balanced plan including both mastery (e.g., washing clothes, showering, and grocery shopping) and pleasurable (e.g., meeting with a friend, reading a book, and engaging in a hobby) events. The previous session focused on pleasant activities that help buffer stress. This session will also add mastery activities to the patient's schedule. The following dialogue can be used to explain the rationale for activity scheduling:

Activity scheduling is an important strategy that can be used to enhance your mood. When someone is depressed, he may be more likely to stay in bed and less likely to engage in a regular schedule of activities. Right? Well, this restriction of activity is likely to contribute to that person feeling even more depressed. The goal of activity scheduling is to devise a plan that allows a gradual reintroduction of regular activity, including both responsibility-based and fun activities.

Use the remainder of session to assist the patient in generating at least one idea for each category (pleasant, mastery). Have the patient consider some of the activities that he used to enjoy or would like to do and record them on the My Activities List in the workbook. Review the Pleasant Events List he circled in Session 2 for ideas. For mastery activities, have the patient think of responsibilities he would like to take on again.

Session Summary

Take a few minutes to review with the patient the most salient points of today's session. It is helpful to consolidate the information and make sure that the patient understands and remembers the important points.

Homework

✎ Have the patient continue to use the Thought Record to monitor thoughts and feelings on a daily basis. This week he will also complete the evaluation column to challenge his negative thinking.

✎ Have the patient continue to add pleasurable and mastery activities to the My Activities List in the workbook.

✎ Have the patient continue to monitor daily activities using the Weekly Activity Schedule.

Chapter 7

Session 5: Cognitive Restructuring—Part III

(Corresponds to chapter 5 of the workbook)

Materials Needed

- Thought Record
- Weekly Activity Schedule

Outline

- Set agenda
- Review Mood Chart
- Review homework
- Assist the patient with generating alternative thoughts to faulty cognitions
- Evaluate consequences and enhance coping for accurate negative cognitions
- Help the patient plan both mastery and pleasurable activities
- Summarize session
- Assign homework

Set Agenda

Open the session with review of the patient's Mood Chart and response to homework combined with information on the general topics to be covered, incorporating the patient's agenda items with those in this manual. (See Session 2 for more instructions on agenda setting.)

Therapist Note

■ *Problem solving applied either formally (Chapter 17) or informally should be considered whenever the patient describes a relevant problematic situation.* ■

Mood Chart Review

Review symptom levels since the previous session using the patient's Mood Chart. Discuss with the patient her attitudes toward symptoms, evaluating the presence of dysfunctional cognitions about moods. Discuss any episodes of medication noncompliance using the medication noncompliance protocol (see Chapter 2).

Homework Review

Homework review should begin with a reminder of what was discussed in the last session. Follow-up questions should focus on difficulties with challenging thoughts using the Thought Record and balancing mastery and pleasurable events on the My Activities List. Review the patient's daily activity level (see Weekly Activity Schedule) and assess cognitions surrounding these events.

Generating Alternative Responses

As therapy progresses and the patient becomes more adept at catching dysfunctional thoughts, there is a greater focus on guiding the patient toward more adaptive thinking strategies. The next step in cognitive restructuring is generating alternative interpretations or responses to faulty cognitions. That is, should the patient lack evidence supporting her thoughts, alternative explanations are considered. The idea is not to generate hyperpositive responses to faulty cognitions, but through challenging a thought, to come up with a more reasonable or likely interpretation. For example, if the patient's initial thought is "I am not good at anything I do," and she is able to generate evidence against this, then a reasonable alternative response may be "There are *some* things that I don't do well, just as there are things that I am able to do well." An unreasonable alternative response would be "I am great at everything that I do."

Assist the patient with generating alternative thoughts or interpretations in response to several examples of distorted thinking from her previous week's Thought Record. Have the patient consider that her initial way of viewing the situation is only one way of looking at it, and help her explore other ways of looking at the situation. Then, encourage the patient to reexamine her mood after considering alternative interpretations. (Use the final column of the Thought Record to document changes in mood.)

The following vignette illustrates the use of Socratic questioning to help the patient consider alternative conceptualizations.

Case Vignette

T: Okay now that you have been successful at identifying thoughts and feelings, and providing evidence for and against these thoughts, let's look at some of the situations that you wrote down over the past week. I see there are several automatic thoughts you had over the past week that are associated with your boss firing you and feelings of incompetence.

P: Yeah. She doesn't say hello to me in the hallways anymore, and she also hasn't been giving me any of the big accounts to work on.

T: OK. That is evidence for. What about evidence against?

P: Well, I guess a good sign is that I just moved into a new office and I got a raise 6 months ago.

T: Okay. Could there be any other reasons explaining your concerns?

P: I don't have any. There have been several lay-offs in the department recently. I could be next.

T: What might be some other reasons for why she hasn't said hello to you in the hallway lately?

P: She has been very busy. She is working on wrapping up one of the biggest accounts the company has ever had.

T: Good point! She may be too busy to say hello.

P: Yeah her mind is probably in many other places.

T: How about the concern that you haven't been assigned any of the new accounts recently? Are there any other explanations for this happening?

P: Well, I suppose I have been pretty busy with my current accounts.

T: And if you are busy with other accounts?

P: I guess I don't have time for any of the new accounts.

T: When you consider these alternative explanations, what happens to your mood?

P: I am very much relieved. I don't feel as incompetent and down on myself. I am much more hopeful that I won't get fired.

Evaluating Consequences and Enhancing Coping

On the other hand, if the patient's thoughts are supported by reasonable evidence, steps should be taken to evaluate consequences and enhance coping to actual threats if they exist. This process of transitioning to a problem-solving approach is illustrated in the following case vignette.

Case Vignette

T: So, it looks like you were able to generate some evidence for the thought "I am not going to make a deadline at work." If this is the case, what is the worst thing that can happen?

P: Well, I could get fired.

T: And what is the likelihood that you will be fired from your job?

P: I guess that is pretty unlikely because I have been there for several years and they really like me.

T: So it seems pretty unlikely. But, if you did get fired, let's talk about how you might deal with that.

Planning Activities

After reviewing the patient's home practice of proposed activities, the next step is to identify a starting place. As mentioned previously, patients frequently want to begin with activities that are mastery or responsibility based because they are behind in activities of daily living. If this is the case, encourage the patient to pick one mastery and one pleasurable activity to include in her plan for the week. For example, you might suggest:

> I know you feel overwhelmed by all the household chores you need to get caught up on, but it is very important that you also participate in activities that are enjoyable. How about striking a balance and consider adding both chore-based and pleasurable activities?

Instruct the patient to use the Weekly Activity Schedule to plan and document time slots for completing each activity. Discuss when, where, and how the patient will carry out each activity. Assist the patient in identifying potential problems when attempting the task.

Troubleshooting Activity Assignments

Activity assignments provide excellent opportunities for cognitive restructuring. Because you are present at the conceptualization of the activity assignment, you are in an excellent position to help the patient evaluate its completion. Common cognitive errors made by patients include evaluating the assignment's success based on previous levels of functioning and activity. For this problem, it may be helpful to remind the patient to gauge success relative to current levels of functioning. A helpful metaphor to illustrate this point is that being depressed is like carrying a 100-pound bag on your back. Thus, completing even a small task is an accomplishment. Another example to emphasize gradual improvement toward a goal is to use the metaphor of recovery from surgery. That is, a patient does not immediately bounce out of bed after a major surgery and run a marathon. Rather, she must approach recovery in a step-by-step fashion (e.g., sitting up, standing, and walking short distances).

In many cases, fuller cognitive restructuring may be warranted, particularly for distortions in the evaluation of performance (e.g., all-or-nothing thinking). For example, in completing a household task (e.g., painting the porch), the patient may have thoughts such as "I must complete it perfectly; if not, I am a failure." Moreover, in carrying out a pleasurable task (e.g., attending a party), the patient may have thoughts such as "I should be the life of the party" or "If I don't talk more, people will not like me." Consequently, before assigning activities, it is useful to devote session time to discussing negative thoughts that may be associated with particular activities and assisting the patient in challenging these thoughts.

The following case example involves a patient who has negative thoughts concerning her activity assignment to spend more time with others. The sections that follow this example illustrate different strategies for challenging these negative thoughts.

Case Vignette

P: I know you said enjoyable activities, like spending time with others, are as important to do as my housework, but I have really had a hard time being around people when I am depressed.

T: What about it is hard for you?

P: I am not really sure. It is so draining when I get together with people. The outings always seem like disasters, and I come home feeling worse about myself than when I left.

T: What happens that makes these situations seem like disasters?

P: Well, it is usually something I do or don't do. I say something that is stupid, or I sit like a bump on a log and don't say anything. Then, everyone at the party thinks I am weird. I go home feeling awful about myself.

Strategy 1: Socratic Questioning

T: How do you know they think you are weird?

P: Well, I am not sure. If you saw someone at a party not saying much to people wouldn't you think they were a little weird?

T: I think there are numerous reasons for why someone might not be talking at a party.

P: Yeah. Like what?

T: Let's reverse the situation. When you are at a party, what do you think about people who are not talking that much?

P: To be honest, I don't spend much time thinking about it. I am not sure I even notice how much each person talks.

T: Is it possible then that people at these parties aren't noticing how much you are talking either?

P: I suppose so.

T: So it is possible that fewer people than you think are drawing conclusions about you?

P: Yeah, I guess that is probably true.

Strategy 2: Use of an Objective Standard

T: Do you still get invitations to parties?

P: Yes.

T: I wonder why people who think you are so weird keep inviting you back.

P: I am not sure. I bet they will eventually stop inviting me.

T: They haven't yet, right?

P: No.

T: So what might that mean?

P: Maybe there is something that I am doing at those parties that they like.

Strategy 3: Role-Play Behavioral Experiment

P: I never have anything interesting to say at these parties anyway.

T: Let's take a minute and test that notion.

P: What do you mean?

T: Let's pretend that you are at a party. I will play the role of someone you meet. Let's have a conversation as if you were really at this party.

After role-playing a party conversation in session, the therapist gives the patient positive feedback about performance and asks her what she thought about her performance. There are occasions in an example like this that a deficiency in social skills or social anxiety may contribute to the patient's not performing well in social situations. Assess for such issues and consider addressing those issues at another point in treatment, mainly in Phase 3.

Strategy 4: Home-Practice Behavioral Experiment

P: I can never finish any household task that I begin. I will never get anything done at home as long as I am depressed!

T: How certain are you that you won't accomplish anything at home?

P: I am 100% certain!

T: You sound pretty sure of yourself. Would you be willing to conduct an experiment and test that prediction over the next week?

P: I could try.

Carefully plan the experiment with the patient. For example, help the patient decide exactly what she is going to do and when she is going to attempt it. Ensure that the task is manageable to increase likelihood of success.

T: What household task would you like to work on?

P: Well, I really want to get the whole house vacuumed. There is dirt everywhere.

T: Are there particular rooms that are more important to you to have vacuumed?

P: I suppose the living room, dining room, and kitchen. They are the rooms with the most traffic and dirt.

T: OK. Why don't you try to do one of those rooms only?

P: How about the kitchen? It is the room that needs it the most.

T: OK. During the next week, I would like you to spend some time cleaning the kitchen. Now, when you go to clean the kitchen, you will be met by all sorts of thoughts telling you that you can't. But I want you to keep in mind that there is a big difference between a thought (which is a guess about how things will go, and, in the case of depression, a very pessimistic guess at that) and behavior. Even though you may have lots of thoughts about how you just can't clean the kitchen, I would like you to go ahead and start and clean for at least 10 minutes. You can go longer, but I want you to at least clean for 10 minutes. Does this sound like something you can do?

P: I guess so.

T: OK, which day do you want to set aside to make your first "push" to clean for 10 minutes?

P: Uh, I should probably try to do it on Thursday.

T: OK, I am going to send you out to test the notion that you can't ever complete a task that you set out to do. I look forward to hearing how it went next week, but I do want you to give me some details about your work. Pay attention to how long you worked and the details of what you got done. OK?

Upon patient's return next session and review of home practice:

T: So how did your experiment go?

P: Well, I cleaned the kitchen floor. It may not have been the best job I have ever done, but I did it!

T: So now what do you think about your idea that you can never get *anything* done while you are depressed?

P: Well, I guess I am not so certain of that anymore. I would say that my percent rating dropped to at least a 50. There are some things that I can get done; it's just that I have to push myself a bit more.

T: That sounds like a fair statement. You have all sorts of negative thoughts about how you can't do anything. But a much more accurate version is that you can do things, but that it is naturally harder because of the feelings of depression. So that you are not ruled by unduly pessimistic thoughts, it will be important for you to use this more accurate thought when you coach yourself about daily events.

Session Summary

Take a few minutes to review with the patient the most salient points of today's session. It is helpful to consolidate the information and make sure that the patient understands and remembers the important points.

Homework

✎ Instruct the patient to participate in at least two planned activities (one mastery and one pleasurable) and complete the Weekly Activity Schedule.

✎ Have the patient complete a Thought Record for the week, adding alternative responses and subsequent changes in feeling state.

Chapter 8 | *Session 6: Cognitive Restructuring—Part III*

(Corresponds to chapter 5 of the workbook)

Materials Needed

- Thought Record
- Weekly Activity Schedule

Outline

- Set agenda
- Review Mood Chart
- Review homework
- Maintain patient use of Thought Records
- Maintain patient use of Weekly Activity Schedule
- Summarize session
- Assign homework

Set Agenda

Open the session with review of the patient's Mood Chart and response to homework combined with information on the general topics to be covered, incorporating the patient's agenda items with those in this manual. (See Session 2 for more instructions on agenda setting.)

Therapist Note

- *Problem solving applied either formally (Chapter 17) or informally should be considered whenever the patient describes a relevant problematic situation.* ■

Mood Chart Review

Review symptom levels since the previous session using the patient's Mood Chart. Discuss with the patient his attitudes toward symptoms, evaluating the presence of dysfunctional cognitions about moods. Discuss any episodes of medication noncompliance using the medication noncompliance protocol (see Chapter 2).

Homework Review

Homework review should begin with a reminder of what was discussed in the last session. Follow-up questions should focus on any difficulties generating alternative thoughts and using all columns of the Thought Record. Review the entire thought-monitoring process with the patient using situations from his homework. It is important to place emphasis on the final step in the Thought Record (evaluating changes in feeling state as a result of altered thinking).

Next, discuss the patient's involvement in activities that were planned as home practice. You may want to ask the following questions:

- *"Did you engage in the agreed upon activities?"*

- *"What difficulties arose, if any?"*

- *"How did you feel after participating in these activities?"*

- *"Did participation in these planned activities have any impact on your overall activity level for the week?"* (Compare this week's activity monitoring form to previous forms.)

Maintaining the Use of Thought Records

The purpose here is to extend the use of the Thought Record concept beyond the session and assigned home practice. You want to encourage the patient to use this format for monitoring and modifying his thoughts on a regular basis. Use of the actual record should be encouraged for several more weeks to ensure that the patient is considering all aspects of cognitive restructuring. Continued use of the Thought Record will also be useful during core belief work in Sessions 7 through 9. Once there is evidence that the patient is able to identify thoughts and feelings, challenge thoughts, and provide alternative explanations without writing the information down, formal use of the Thought Record can be faded out. You might address this point by saying:

> *As I said before, you really seem to have the hang of cognitive restructuring. Given that it has been a helpful strategy for you, it is important to keep up the momentum of using this skill on a regular basis. Therefore, I suggest that you continue to use the actual Thought Record for a few more weeks or so. In a sense, I am asking you to over practice the concept of recording and challenging your thoughts. The more practice you get now, the easier it will be for you to incorporate a new style of thinking into your daily life. After some additional practice, you can fade out the use of the actual recording form. At that point, I hope you will find yourself going through cognitive restructuring steps in your mind when you sense a change in your mood state. Does this all sound reasonable to you?*

Get feedback from the patient. You may also want to mention that in the next few sessions the use of the Thought Record will come in handy to learn a new concept—core beliefs.

Maintaining the Use of Activity Schedules

A rationale similar to that of continuing the use of the Thought Record applies to continued use of the Weekly Activity Schedule. The ongoing use of an activity schedule for monitoring and planning daily activities is recommended. Remind the patient that information on the Weekly Activity Schedule (e.g., decreased level of involvement) can serve as an indicator that a more severe depression may be imminent. It can also serve as a device for planning and following through with scheduled events. Encourage the patient to complete the Weekly Activity Schedule every evening. Throughout the remainder of the sessions, check in with the patient about his ongoing use of this strategy. Eventually, a modified version of the activity schedule can be devised to assist the patient in maintaining a higher level of interaction with the environment.

Session Summary

Take a few minutes to review with the patient the most salient points of today's session. It is helpful to consolidate the information and make sure that the patient understands and remembers the important points.

Homework

✎ Have the patient continue to use Thought Records for modifying thoughts.

✎ Have the patient add at least two activities (one mastery and one pleasurable) and continue daily monitoring of events using the Weekly Activity Schedule.

Chapter 9

Session 7: Core Beliefs

(Corresponds to chapter 6 of the workbook)

Materials Needed

- Core Belief Worksheet

Outline

- Set agenda

- Review Mood Chart

- Review homework

- Help the patient identify core beliefs

- Introduce the Core Belief Worksheet

- Educate the patient about the nature of core beliefs

- Assess ongoing activity goals

- Summarize session

- Assign homework

Set Agenda

Open the session with review of the patient's Mood Chart and response to homework combined with information on the general topics to be covered, incorporating the patient's agenda items with those in this manual. (See Session 2 for more instructions on agenda setting.)

Review Mood Chart

Review symptom levels since the previous session using the patient's Mood Chart. Discuss with the patient her attitudes toward symptoms, evaluating the presence of dysfunctional cognitions about moods. Discuss any episodes of medication noncompliance using the medication non-compliance protocol (see Chapter 2).

Homework Review

Homework review should begin with a reminder of what was discussed in the last session. Review the patient's Thought Record and Weekly Activity Schedule. Follow-up questions should focus on any difficulties modifying thoughts and engaging in activities. If necessary, problem solve difficulties with the patient.

Introduction to Core Beliefs

Core beliefs involve an individual's most central ideas about the self and are often formed early in life. Frequently, core beliefs revolve around themes of unlovability or incompetence/helplessness. Core beliefs in the unlovability domain may involve themes of being defective or undesirable. Core beliefs in the incompetence or helplessness domain may involve themes of personal vulnerability or weakness. Alternatively, such core beliefs may revolve around themes of failure or disrespect in areas of achievement.

In acutely depressed patients, core beliefs are often activated and accessible. Depressed patients may readily state "I feel that no one will ever love me" or "I don't think that I will ever succeed at anything." However, identifying and challenging core beliefs is a crucial strategy not only in the treatment of acute depression, but also in the prevention of relapse.

Throughout the progression of therapy and cognitive restructuring work, you may have a sense of a general theme or themes underlying the patient's dysfunctional thoughts. Nonetheless, it is important for you to explore hunches with the patient and share conceptualizations with her before drawing final conclusions. One way to reach the level of core beliefs is by asking the patient the following questions:

- *"What was the meaning of that thought?"*

- *"What do you think it was about that particular event or situation that got you so upset?"*

It is always important to present core beliefs in an exploratory, collaborative way rather than to definitively state the patient's vulnerabilities, thereby avoiding or minimizing defensiveness. Alternatively, you may ask the patient if she can observe a general theme or themes in her dysfunctional thoughts. The following vignette illustrates how to progress from the level of in-the-moment automatic thoughts to core beliefs:

Case Vignette

T: So, at what times during the week did you feel the most depressed?

P: Um . . . probably when I was sitting alone in my apartment.

T: Do you recall what types of thoughts you were having when you felt the most depressed?

P: Well, I was having thoughts like "I will never find anyone again. Steve dumped me and no one will ever want me."

T: Why do you think that no one else would ever want you?

P: Well, Steve began to dislike certain things about me once he really got to know me.

T: What does that mean to you that he began to dislike certain things about you?

P: Well, I guess it means that there is something very wrong with me and that I will never really find someone who loves me.

T: It seems to me that a common theme in the situations that we have discussed over the last several weeks involves the belief that you are unlovable or undesirable in some way. What do you think about that?

What are Core Beliefs?

The goal is to educate the patient about the nature of core beliefs and their relationship to automatic thoughts. The discussion may begin as follows:

> *These general themes in your automatic thoughts are also known as "core beliefs." Your core beliefs may have been formed early in your life and they may affect the way that you view yourself and the world around you. For example, the belief "I'm unlovable" is what we call a core belief. These types of negative beliefs may be dormant during times when you are feeling well and activated when you get depressed. When depressed, your core belief may act as a filter. For example, all of the information that supports the negative belief may readily filter through. However, any evidence contradicting the negative belief may be ignored or discounted. These types of negative beliefs can contribute to getting depressed, particularly when negative events happen that relate to your core belief.*

Give some examples of patient's negative beliefs. Explain that when the patient accepts these negative beliefs as "truths" about herself, it also makes it difficult to feel better and to fight the depression. The goal of the next three sessions is to help her discover some of her core beliefs, the impact that these self-views may be having on maintaining her depression, and strategies for challenging these long-standing beliefs. Ask the patient if she has any questions thus far.

At this point, the patient may ask about the differences between core beliefs and the automatic thoughts she has been working on over the past several weeks. Stress the idea that core beliefs typically relate to underlying themes across various situations and automatic thoughts. Additionally, core beliefs typically have been present for many years.

At the conclusion of the session, ask the patient to summarize the general themes in the automatic thoughts she has noted thus far. Encourage her to monitor her thoughts during the week, attempting to identify underlying core beliefs. The Core Belief Worksheet in the workbook is designed to help patients with this exercise. A copy for your use is provided in the appendix.

Weekly Activity Levels

Before closing the session with summaries, check in with the patient on activity goals. Assess whether the patient is continuing to pursue weekly pleasurable activities at a reasonable level. Assign additional activities as needed.

Session Summary

Take a few minutes to review with the patient the most salient points of today's session. It is helpful to consolidate the information and make sure that the patient understands and remembers the important points.

Homework

✎ Instruct the patient to continue using the Thought Record to monitor automatic thoughts and examine these thoughts further to determine underlying core beliefs.

✎ Encourage the patient to apply knowledge from the Thought Record to completing the Core Belief Worksheet.

✎ Have the patient continue to monitor daily activities using the Weekly Activity Schedule.

Chapter 10 | *Session 8: Challenging Core Beliefs*

(Corresponds to chapter 7 of the workbook)

Materials Needed

- Core Belief Worksheet

Outline

- Set agenda

- Review Mood Chart

- Review homework

- Help the patient identify and challenge core beliefs

- Work with the patient to find intermediate beliefs

- Discuss the origins of core beliefs referring to childhood experiences

- Summarize session

- Assign homework

Set Agenda

Open the session with review of the patient's Mood Chart and response to homework combined with information on the general topics to be covered, incorporating the patient's agenda items with those in this manual. (See Session 2 for more instructions on agenda setting.)

Mood Chart Review

Review symptom levels since the previous session using the patient's Mood Chart. Discuss with the patient his attitudes toward symptoms, evaluating the presence of dysfunctional cognitions about moods. Discuss any episodes of medication noncompliance using the medication noncompliance protocol (see Chapter 2).

Homework Review

Discussion should focus on a review of general themes of automatic thoughts, use of the Core Belief Worksheet, and any difficulties that arose in identifying core beliefs that underlie automatic thoughts. Also, continue to check-in on scheduled activities and use of the Weekly Activity Schedule.

Identifying and Challenging Core Beliefs

Depending on how readily accessible the core beliefs were in the last session, you may need to spend more time in this session discussing general themes and formulating hypotheses about core beliefs. After core beliefs have been identified, it is important to proceed to strategies for challenging them.

Explain that the patient can challenge core beliefs in much the same way he has been taught to challenge his automatic thoughts. Remind the patient that individuals, especially when depressed, have a tendency to view their beliefs as facts. Furthermore, they tend to look for support to back up these faulty beliefs. Set the stage for the patient to generate support contrary to his belief to turn off or modify the filtration system that he has been using. The following case vignette (where the core belief "I am incompetent" has been identified) demonstrates this process.

Case Vignette

T: Core beliefs such as this one may act as a filter or a screen when you get depressed. For example, over the past several weeks, it seems that all of the information supporting the idea "I'm incompetent" has readily filtered through. However, it seems that any evidence supporting the idea that you are competent has been ignored or negated. Can you think of any situations that support the idea that you are competent?

P: Well, I guess I have been doing all right in some of my classes.

T: Do you consider that as evidence that you are competent?

P: Well, the classes I am referring to are fairly straightforward. I should be able to do OK in those.

T: Do you think that this way of viewing your performance in classes is being filtered by your core belief?

P: Well, I guess, maybe it is. Come to think of it, some of my classmates have had difficulties in those classes and have asked me for help.

Finding Intermediate Beliefs

In restructuring core beliefs, often it is important to find intermediate beliefs that the patient is willing to accept. For example, it is unlikely that a patient will jump from feeling completely inadequate to completely adequate. An intermediate step might be "I am reasonably adequate at many things." Work with the patient in this session to find an intermediate belief that he may be willing to accept.

Core Beliefs and Childhood Experiences

A crucial part of understanding and modifying core beliefs may involve identifying the developmental and historical precursors of the core beliefs. In this session, begin this discussion by asking the patient the following questions:

- *"Do you recall when you first felt* (the core belief, e.g., incompetent or unlovable)*?"*

- *"Were there any times in your childhood when you felt this way?"*

Occasionally, the development of core beliefs is readily understood by both patient and therapist. For example, some patients who have suffered emotional or physical abuse may readily cite situations in which they first recall endorsing the core belief. However, the development of core beliefs may often be more subtle and require some exploration. For example, perhaps a child had the experience of never quite fitting in with peers, and developed the belief "I'm different" or "I'm defective." A child who had been compared to an older sibling may have developed the belief "I don't measure up" or "I'm incompetent."

Recovering this information can often be helpful because children typically believe information that they are given. By viewing this information retrospectively as an adult, the patient can begin to question the veracity or fairness of the messages that he came to believe about himself as a child. This may be explained to the patient in the following way:

> As children, we tend to believe what we are told. In a way, children
> are like sponges, they absorb what is given to them by their
> environment. This type of learning can occur in the context of direct
> messages that we receive from authority figures (parents, teachers, etc.)
> or from peers. However, sometimes this type of learning occurs more
> subtly. Sometimes negative messages are given to us unfairly as children
> and we come to believe these as truths. For this reason, I would like to
> try to explore with you how you developed these beliefs about yourself.
> And then, perhaps, we can test out these messages to see if it is really
> fair or true to apply these beliefs to yourself as an adult. Does that
> sound okay to you?

Occasionally, it may be difficult for the patient to understand this concept as it applies to him. Just as in the coaching story from Session 2, it may be easier to convey this concept of identifying and challenging core beliefs using a story about someone else. You may use the following story about Mr. J. to illustrate the importance of examining the historical context of the core belief.

Case Example

Mr. J. had always held the belief that he was inferior and incompetent, particularly in areas related to school and work achievement. The youngest of three brothers, he had relative difficulty in school and was often compared to his older brothers by his parents. He recalls having difficulty in math skills and feeling humiliated by this inadequacy. While he performed relatively well in high school and graduated from a state college, he still felt like a relative failure in contrast to his two older brothers, who graduated from Ivy League schools and pursued law school, like their father. Mr. J. performed well in his job selling life insurance and was well liked by his boss and coworkers. However, when he became depressed, his core beliefs of inadequacy tended to resurface, leaving him doubtful about his abilities and discouraged about his financial situation. Although, he was happily married and owned a home in a pleasant, middle-class neighborhood, he would begin to compare himself to his brothers, who were wealthier and held more prestigious positions in law firms. When depressed, he would also doubt his abilities at work, withdrawing from sales meetings and reducing his client contact. Paradoxically, such behaviors resulted in lower sales figures for the month, further confirming his core beliefs of inadequacy.

An intervention used with Mr. J. involved his view of his own son who was currently in 4th grade (around the same age as Mr. J. was when he developed his core belief of inadequacy). When questioned about how he would treat his son if he had difficulties in school, he began to realize for the first time that he had been treated unfairly. He began to realize that he had skills that his older brothers did not have. However, his parents did not praise those skills and talents (sports, good social skills, etc). Mr. J. began to recognize and evaluate how his core beliefs still pushed him around today. He learned to value some of his talents and to judge himself against his own standards.

Revisiting the Core Belief Worksheet

After obtaining childhood data from the patient, revisit the Core Belief Worksheet with the patient, noting how childhood experiences contributed to the development of the core belief.

Session Summary

Take a few minutes to review with the patient the most salient points of today's session. It is helpful to consolidate the information and make sure that the patient understands and remembers the important points.

Homework

✎ Instruct the patient to continue using the Thought Record to monitor automatic thoughts, and examine these thoughts further to determine underlying core beliefs. Use of the Thought Record should be done with sensitivity to identifying automatic thoughts related to the beliefs noted on the Core Belief Worksheet.

✎ Have the patient continue to monitor daily activities using the Weekly Activity Schedule.

Chapter 11 | *Session 9: More Work With Core Beliefs*

(Corresponds to chapter 8 of the workbook)

Materials Needed

- Thought Record

Outline

- Set agenda
- Review Mood Chart
- Review homework
- Explore the patient's core beliefs as triggers for worsening mood
- Help the patient readjust expectations
- Summarize session
- Assign homework

Set Agenda

Open the session with review of the patient's Mood Chart and response to homework combined with information on the general topics to be covered, incorporating the patient's agenda items with those in this manual. (See Session 2 for more instructions on agenda setting.)

Mood Chart Review

Review symptom levels since the previous session using the patient's Mood Chart. Discuss with the patient her attitudes toward symptoms, evaluating the presence of dysfunctional cognitions about moods. Discuss any episodes of medication noncompliance using the medication noncompliance protocol (see Chapter 2).

Homework Review

Refer back to the patient's completed Thought Record, and review typical situations that occurred during the week. Pay special attention to those situations in which the patient noted that her core belief was filtering her experience. Review the childhood data obtained from the previous session and inquire if the patient has viewed her core belief with a slightly different perspective. Stress that with practice core beliefs change gradually over time. Check if the patient was able to adopt some intermediate steps in reformulating the core belief.

Also, continue to check in on scheduled activities and use of the Weekly Activity Schedule.

Core Beliefs as Triggers for Worsening Mood

In this session, begin to discuss the idea of core beliefs as particular areas of vulnerability. In other words, individuals are more likely to respond negatively to a situation if it has special meaning for them. Explore with the patient the types of triggers that have precipitated episodes in the past and discuss how these situations may have been related to patient's core beliefs. Such vulnerabilities are important targets of intervention in both the treatment of acute depression and relapse prevention. In addition to modifying negative core beliefs, problem-solving efforts should focus on situations that are relevant to the patient's specific areas of vulnerability.

The triggers for a depressive episode may differ depending on the nature of an individual's core beliefs. Some individuals place great value on being accepted and loved by others. These individuals may be devastated by losses or rejections in the interpersonal domain. A typical belief endorsed by such an individual may be "I am nothing if others do not love me." Others place the greatest value on the need for independence or freedom from control. Such individuals may exhibit high levels of self-criticism, particularly with regard to achievement domains. Such individuals may fear setbacks at work or criticisms of their abilities and may be most vulnerable to situations revealing perceived areas of incompetence.

Again, if the patient has difficulty relating to this personally, you may return to the case example of Mr. J. to illustrate this point. You can summarize the following information in the case material that follows. This case also illustrates that episodes of depression can contribute to behaviors which seem to sustain or confirm the core belief. On the Core Belief Worksheet, these behaviors are labeled "Core Strategies." Devote time in the session to helping the patient identify which behaviors may be used to defend against, and may also maintain core beliefs (e.g., rejecting others before they reject you, or leaving a social or work situation). These types of behaviors should be a top priority for change, with rehearsal of useful alternative behaviors.

Case Example

Treatment for Mr. J. was about modifying his core beliefs of inadequacy and helping him target those specific behaviors that served to confirm his core beliefs (e.g., avoiding work responsibilities when depressed). For example, Mr. J. and his therapist targeted specific ways for him to stay on track with clients when feeling depressed. While Mr. J. was usually highly motivated to pursue meetings with clients, he and his therapist acknowledged his tendency to withdraw from clients when depressed. In addition to challenging interfering negative thoughts, he set up a system in which he tracked his number of sales calls per day and discussed this each week during therapy. In this way, he was able to keep his core beliefs from becoming a self-fulfilling prophecy.

Readjusting Expectations

In bipolar patients, core beliefs may be directly related to beliefs about their illness. For example, bipolar patients may have powerful "evidence" to support negative beliefs about themselves. Some patients may have been abandoned by spouses, friends, or family members because of behaviors when manic or depressed. Others may have suffered acute losses in their careers. Some students may have dropped out of school or missed semesters due to severe episodes. Along with modifying core beliefs, the work of therapy involves helping patients readjust their personal expectations toward step-by-step goal attainment from their current state. Effort in cognitive restructuring is accordingly devoted to identifying "should" statements in relation to life stages (e.g., "I should own a house by now." "I should be through with school now."), as well as over-effort that is part of trying to "make up for lost time." Make clear to the patient that trying to make up for lost time enhances anxiety, tension, and negative affect. The alternative goal is to empathically accept that the bipolar disorder has disrupted life plans, but to continue a focus on the next reasonable goal given current life circumstances. Work with the patient to complete the Long-Term Goal Sheet in Chapter 8 of the workbook (a copy for your reference is provided in the appendix). Additional information on this process can be found in *Living with Bipolar Disorder: A Guide for Individuals and Families* (Otto et al., 2008, Oxford University Press).

Session Summary

Take a few minutes to review with the patient the most salient points of today's session. It is helpful to consolidate the information and make sure that the patient understands and remembers the important points.

Homework

  Have the patient continue to monitor and challenge core beliefs, and explore intermediate beliefs using the Thought Record and, as needed, the Core Belief Worksheet.

✎ Instruct the patient to target behaviors that sustain the core belief.

✎ Have the patient note three typical situations that may be likely to trigger dysfunctional cognitions related to core beliefs to aid early identification of dysfunctional cognitive patterns. Engage in problem solving about alternative cognitive and behavioral responses to these situations.

✎ Have patient continue to schedule activities and monitor these on the Weekly Activity Schedule.

Treatment Phase 2

Chapter 12 | *Session 10: Drafting a Treatment Contract*

(Corresponds to chapter 9 of the workbook)

Materials Needed

- Treatment Contract

Outline

- Set agenda

- Review Mood Chart

- Review homework

- Introduce Treatment Contract and rationale for use

- Review components of Treatment Contract

- Discuss selection of support team members

- Discuss involvement of support members in the next couple of sessions

- Summarize session

- Assign homework

Set Agenda

Open the session with review of the patient's Mood Chart and response to homework combined with information on the general topics to be covered, incorporating the patient's agenda items with those in this manual. (See Session 2 for more instructions on agenda setting.)

Mood Chart Review

Review symptom levels since the previous session using the patient's Mood Chart. Discuss with the patient his attitudes toward symptoms, evaluating the presence of dysfunctional cognitions about moods. Discuss any episodes of medication noncompliance using the medication noncompliance protocol (see Chapter 2).

Homework Review

Review outcome of patient's monitoring and challenging core beliefs. Discuss with the patient alternative responses for situations that are high risk for eliciting negative core beliefs and associated behaviors. Discuss any difficulties the patient experienced in implementing the restructuring or problem-solving assignments.

Also, continue to check on scheduled activities and use of the Weekly Activity Schedule.

Introduction to Treatment Contract and Rationale for Use

Refer the patient to the Treatment Contract in Chapter 9 of the workbook and review its purpose and contents. Stress to the patient that using the Treatment Contract is an important step in managing his bipolar disorder. Explain that the Treatment Contract provides an opportunity for the patient to plan in advance for detecting early signs of hypomania and depression and preventing/coping with full-blown episodes. In addition to documenting his symptoms, this process involves selecting and educating a support system that will participate with him on his Treatment Contract. This support system may include doctors, family members, spouse or significant other, friends, coworkers, etc.

It is important that the patient's support system receive information about bipolar disorder. They can obtain and read a copy of *Living with Bipolar Disorder: A Guide for Individuals and Families* (Otto et al., 2008, Oxford University Press), or they can read the patient's treatment workbook. Friends and family should also ask the patient about his specific symptoms. The patient may also invite any members of his support system to attend some of his upcoming sessions. Explain that in order to involve the patient's support system, he must specify ways in which they can be helpful to him during acute episodes. He may also wish to give permission to his support system to contact his treatment team when they detect impending symptoms of mania and depression.

The story of Homer's Odysseus can be used to illustrate the rationale for the Treatment Contract.

Odysseus and the Sirens

You may remember that Odysseus and his crew were lost at sea and spent many years returning to their homeland. During their years of travel, they experienced a number of adventures. One adventure concerned their travel near the island of the sirens. The sirens were women who would sing songs that were so beautiful that sailors would be lured too close and wreck upon the treacherous rocks surrounding the island. Odysseus wanted to hear the song of the sirens, but knew he could not trust himself to keep the ship safe. Therefore, Odysseus used his powers as captain of the ship to prevent a disaster. He instructed his crew, "On hearing the sirens' song, pour wax in your ears and bind me to the mast of the ship. If I protest, bind me even tighter." Odysseus used his power as captain to make sure that his crew prevented him from causing harm to the ship.

In a similar way, you can empower your crew, or support system, by instructing them to anticipate problems and informing them of the types of reactions and responses you would prefer them to make. By designing the Treatment Contract, you act as the "captain of your ship" and instruct your crew to react to the challenges anticipated in the course of the journey. By planning ahead when you are feeling relatively well, you maintain maximal control and power and reduce the risk of people imposing unwanted restrictions on you if you experience a full-blown episode.

Components of Treatment Contract

After discussing the rationale, look at the contract and review the format with the patient. A copy of the contract can be found on page 123.

You may use the following sample dialogue:

First, you must recognize that you have bipolar disorder. Then, you need to specify the members of your support team.

Next, you will specify how you know you are well. You do this by mapping out a plan for your euthymic periods, stating what your goals are and what things you would like to accomplish when in a stable mood state.

Second, you specify thoughts, feelings, behaviors, and early warning signs for your episodes of depression. That is, those symptoms that best reflect your experience of depression. Next, you specify a plan for coping with depression, stating ways in which your support system can be helpful to you.

Third, you note the thoughts, feelings, and behaviors and early warning signs of hypomania and mania. Just as you did for depression, you will specify a plan for coping with mania or hypomania, giving specific instructions to the members of your support system in this plan. It is often your family or support system who will first recognize the signs of mania. You may also want to specify who initiates the plan for mania. Do you have any questions?

Treatment Contract

The purpose of this contract is to organize my care for bipolar disorder, with attention to both the prevention of mood episodes and the efficient treatment of these episodes should they occur. My first step in guiding my care is the selection of my support team. The team members should include people with whom I have regular contact, who can help me identify episodes should they occur and help me put into practice some of the tools I have learned in treatment.

My second step in developing this contract is to identify tools I will use to help control my bipolar disorder so that I can best pursue my life goals.

Check
Intent to Use

_____ **Monitor my mood for early intervention.**

I know from my own mood patterns that I should watch out for the following signs:

Depressed Thoughts _____

_____

Depressed Symptoms _____

_____

Depressed Behavior _____

_____

Hypomanic Thoughts _____

_____

Hypomanic Symptoms _____

_____

Hypomanic Behaviors _____

_____

_____ **Take early action if I notice signs of depression or mania.**

_____ Contact my psychiatrist at phone #_____.

_____ Contact my therapist at phone #_____.

_____ Contact my support person at phone #_____.

_____ Maintain a regular schedule of sleep and activities.

_____ Maintain a regular schedule of pleasant events.

continued

_____ Evaluate my thoughts for negative or hyperpositive thinking.

_____ Talk with my family about ways to cope.

_____ Limit my alcohol use and avoid all non-medication drugs.

_____ Other _____.

_____ Other _____.

_____ Other _____.

_____ Other _____.

_____ **Take active steps to keep my mood in the desired range:**

_____ Take all medications as prescribed by my doctor.

_____ Maintain regular appointments with my psychiatrist at ------/month.

_____ Maintain regular appointments with my therapist at ------/month.

_____ Keep a regular sleep schedule.

_____ Maintain a schedule including at least 3 valued activities each day as a buffer against stress.

_____ Avoid excessive use of alcohol.

_____ Avoid all use of illicit drugs.

_____ Use no alcohol for the next 30 days

_____ Use no recreational drugs for the next 30 days

_____ Keep a perspective on my thoughts, and evaluate my thoughts for accuracy.

_____ Share with my family information on communication styles that may reduce stress.

_____ Other _____.

_____ Other _____.

_____ Other _____.

_____ Other _____.

_____ **Contact the following people should I ever have strong suicidal thoughts:**

_____ Contact my psychiatrist at phone #_____.

_____ Contact my therapist at phone #_____.

continued

_____ Contact my support person at phone #_____.

_____ Other action_____.

_____ **Keep myself safe until I can be seen or go to a local emergency room if I ever fear I may act on suicidal thoughts.**

_____ **If I start to become depressed, I would like my support team to:**

_____ Talk to me about my symptoms (who_____)

_____ Make plans for a pleasant event (who_____)

_____ Discuss ways to reduce stress (who_____)

_____ Make sure I am taking my medication (who_____)

_____ Call my doctor if I am unable to (who_____)

_____ Other _____

_____ Other _____

_____ Other _____

_____ **If I start to become manic, I would like my support team to:**

_____ Talk to me about my symptoms (who_____)

_____ Talk to me about reducing activities (who_____)

_____ Allow me to be alone if I am irritable (who_____)

_____ Take care of the kids/pets/other (who_____)

_____ Take away my credit cards (who_____)

_____ Take away my car keys (who_____)

_____ Take me to the hospital (preferred hospital _____)

_____ Other _____

_____ Other _____

_____ Other _____

I understand that this contract is designed by me so that I can take an active role in my treatment. My goal is to maximize my control by arranging for my support team to take care of me. So that any future decisions are well considered, I agree to change this contract only after giving 2 weeks written notice to all parties to this contract.

Signatures for contracting individuals

_____   _____

Signature   Date   Signature   Date

An important step in using a Treatment Contract is selection of a support team. These team members should be people with whom the patient has regular contact and who can help identify episodes when they occur. There is a form in the workbook that the patient can use to identify members of his support team. The following vignette illustrates how to help a patient determine whom to include as a part of his support network.

Case Vignette

P: So, I've been thinking about this Treatment Contract, and I'm having a little trouble figuring out who to put on the contract.

T: Have you thought about anyone that you would definitely put on the contract?

P: Yeah. My psychiatrist is definitely going to be on it. I showed it to him and he agreed to do it. We figured out how I could get a hold of him if it was an emergency. We also talked about where I'd want to be hospitalized. Some of this stuff we had talked about already, but it was helpful to go over it again. I also put you on the contract. I don't know who else to put on the contract, though. I thought about my mom or my brother, but I don't know. . . . I also thought about asking some of my coworkers?

T: Well, let's think about this. You could simply leave me and your psychiatrist on the contract and that would be a great start. We'll make sure to spend some time talking about what you'd like me to do should you get too high or too low. You could also put others on this contract, so long as you feel comfortable discussing it with them and you would consider them trustworthy. The people you add should be those that see you or at least those that you speak to frequently enough that they will notice any changes in your mood. Also, remember that you'll probably revise this contract over time, so that you can always add people at any time.

P: There's one coworker who I'm really close with that I've already told about my illness. He was pretty supportive the last time that I had some difficulty, and he's also been really good about being discrete with the other people we work with.

T: So, it sounds as though he might be helpful to include on the contract. Have you thought about how he could be included?

P: I think it would be most helpful if he'd let me know if he noticed any changes in my mood. For example, he could let me know if I'm snapping at other people, or if I'm getting too high.

T: That seems like a reasonable plan. Have you mentioned anything to him about this?

P: Not yet. I'm worried that it might be too much of an imposition to ask him to do this.

T: Although that's certainly a valid concern, it might be worth bringing it up with him and getting his feedback about what he might or might not be comfortable doing. Sometimes, friends or relatives are relieved to have a plan in place that they can implement if you are having trouble. It might also be helpful to discuss with him the signs that you are getting depressed or manic and to distinguish those from normal mood changes.

T: Would you be comfortable having him call your psychiatrist or me if he gets concerned about you?

P: I really think that this would be too much for him to do.

T: Alright. Given your concerns about making too many demands on your coworker, I'm wondering if there's anyone else that you would like to put on your contract. Sometimes people find it helpful to have multiple people on their contract so that the responsibility is shared. People can also take on different roles, depending on their availability and willingness to participate.

P: Come to think about it, I don't want to ask my mother. She'd get too worried. I don't want to stress her out. My brother would be cool, though. He knows all about my illness and he was the one who helped me get to the hospital the first time I got sick.

T: So he might also be a good person to include.

P: Yep. I would feel good having him talk to my psychiatrist or to you.

T: OK. Do you see him often?

P: I see him pretty much every week. We get together at my mom's house, or we go out.

T: Again, it would probably be helpful to go over the contract with him to clarify what normal versus depressed versus manic mood looks like for you, and what helpful strategies might be. Do you have an idea of how you would bring this up with him?

P: We're supposed to go to my mother's house for dinner this weekend. That would probably be the best time to talk to him.

T: Great. I would suggest that you bring the contract with you. If you can find some quiet time to go over it with him that would be ideal. Next week, we can discuss how things went with your brother and coworker, and go over any issues that came up.

At the conclusion of the session, if the patient already has some idea of whom he would like to include on the Treatment Contract, encourage him to discuss the contract with those people before the next session. In this case, it is helpful to review with the patient what to discuss with whom and how to present the contract to each member of his support team.

Involvement of Support Members in Sessions

Ask the patient to consider inviting family members and/or members of his support team to the next two sessions. Discuss with the patient the role that the support member will play during these sessions, and any concerns that the patient may have about involving others in sessions.

Session Summary

Take a few minutes to review with the patient the most salient points of today's session. It is helpful to consolidate the information and make sure that the patient understands and remembers the important points.

Homework

✎ Have the patient complete the symptom checklists found in the Treatment Contract documenting depressive, elevated, and euthymic symptoms.

✎ Have the patient consider whom to include on his support team for the Treatment Contract. If prepared to do so, he should discuss the contract with these individuals and their role as a member on the support team.

✎ If prepared to do so, have the patient invite members of his support network to attend upcoming sessions.

Session 11: Drafting a Treatment Contract

(Corresponds to chapter 9 of the workbook)

Materials Needed

- Treatment Contract

Outline

- Set agenda
- Review Mood Chart
- Review homework
- Discuss possible problem areas of the Treatment Contract
- Involve family or support team members in discussion
- Summarize session
- Assign homework

Set Agenda

See previous sessions. If family or support members are in attendance, involve them in collaboratively setting the agenda. Make sure to leave enough time to address their specific concerns or questions and involve them in discussions about the Treatment Contract.

Mood Chart Review

Review symptom levels since the previous session using the patient's Mood Chart. Discuss with the patient her attitudes toward symptoms, evaluating the presence of dysfunctional cognitions about moods. Discuss any episodes of medication noncompliance using the medication noncompliance protocol (see Chapter 2).

Homework Review

Review symptom checklists found in the Treatment Contract documenting depressive, elevated, and euthymic symptoms.

Ask the patient if she has identified whom she would like to include as members of her support team and if she has approached these individuals. Discuss how the presentation of the Treatment Contract went or any concerns she has about approaching potential members. If not at this session, talk about whether any support team members will be joining the next session.

Possible Problem Areas of the Treatment Contract

A problem area frequently discussed by patients includes a sense that the Treatment Contract will limit their freedom or control. Acknowledge this as a common reaction. Encourage the patient to discuss this concern and repeatedly stress the ways in which the contract improves her control and power over bipolar disorder.

Other patients may feel that the contract does not apply to their specific concerns. Encourage the patient to personalize the contract to reflect her individual symptoms and goals. The patient can cross off symptoms that don't apply or write in additional symptoms. The contract can also be rewritten, if necessary.

Family or Support Member Involvement

If a family or support member attends the session, engage them in the discussion about the Treatment Contract. Encourage the patient to discuss how the support member can be involved in the contract. Support members may vary widely in their existing knowledge about bipolar disorder. Make sure to leave enough time to address their specific concerns or questions about bipolar disorder and its treatment.

If the support members are included on the contract, address specific issues regarding communication. Elicit feedback from the patient regarding her preferences for communication between you and the support system member. Ideally, open communication between you and support members works best in facilitating the Treatment Contract. However, occasionally there are certain topics that the patient would like to deem "off limits." A signed "release of information" by the patient covers the therapist's bases in setting these agreements.

Session Summary

Take a few minutes to review with the patient the most salient points of today's session. It is helpful to consolidate the information and make sure that the patient understands and remembers the important points.

Homework

✎ Encourage the patient to continue to develop the Treatment Contract.

✎ Ask the patient to approach and discuss the contract with potential support team members.

✎ Encourage the patient to invite members of her support network to attend upcoming sessions.

(Corresponds to chapter 9 of the workbook)

Materials Needed

- Treatment Contract

Outline

- Set agenda

- Review Mood Chart

- Review homework

- Involve family or support member (if present) in discussion of Treatment Contract

- Define problem areas to be addressed in Sessions 14–20 (Phase 3)

- Summarize session

- Assign homework

Setting the Agenda

See previous sessions. If family or support members are in attendance, involve them in collaboratively setting the agenda. Make sure to leave enough time to address their specific concerns or questions and involve them in discussions about the Treatment Contract and workbook. If the same family or support member was present in the previous session, include issues carried over from the previous session.

Mood Chart Review

Review symptom levels since the previous session using the patient's Mood Chart. Discuss with the patient his attitudes toward symptoms, evaluating the presence of dysfunctional cognitions about moods. Discuss any episodes of medication noncompliance using the medication noncompliance protocol (see Chapter 2).

Homework Review

Check with the patient to see if he has completed the Treatment Contract and discussed it with support team members. Any problems with this should be added to this session's agenda.

Family or Support Member Involvement

If family or support members attend the session, engage them in the discussion about the Treatment Contract. Encourage the patient to discuss how support members can be involved in the contract. Support members may vary widely in their existing knowledge about bipolar disorder. Make sure to leave enough time to address specific concerns or questions about bipolar disorder and its treatment.

Sometimes family or support members may inquire about attending future sessions. While this may be potentially beneficial, this treatment is designed to be an individual therapy. However, further support member attendance would be allowable in situations of acute crisis (e.g., if there is concern over the possibility of an impending suicide attempt or in the presence of erratic manic behavior requiring amendments to the Treatment Contract).

Defining Problem Areas

Work with the patient to develop a list of problem areas and treatment goals that can be targeted in future sessions (Phase 3, Sessions 14–20). These upcoming sessions will utilize a flexible, modular approach allowing for attention to specific areas of difficulty for each patient (see Chapter 16 for more information on the Problem-List Phase of treatment).

Session Summary

Take a few minutes to review with the patient the most salient points of today's session. It is helpful to consolidate the information and make sure that the patient understands and remembers the important points.

Homework

- Have the patient prepare for next session's discussion of mania by reflecting on changes in thoughts, feelings, and behaviors that occurred during previous manic episodes.

- Instruct the patient to make any necessary revisions to the Treatment Contract and have all treatment team members sign it.

Chapter 15

Session 13: Hypomanic Cognitive Errors

(Corresponds to chapter 10 of the workbook)

Materials Needed

- List of hypomanic cognitive errors

- List of strategies to interfere with impulsive, hypomanic behaviors

- Patient's completed Treatment Contract

Outline

- Set agenda

- Review Mood Chart

- Review homework

- Present and discuss hypomanic cognitive errors

- Work through an example of challenging hyperpositive thinking

- Discuss strategies to prevent impulsive, hypomanic behaviors

- Detect problems in implementing prevention strategies

- Summarize session

- Assign homework

Set Agenda

See previous sessions for information on setting the agenda.

Mood Chart Review

Review symptom levels since the previous session using the patient's Mood Chart. Discuss with the patient her attitudes toward symptoms, evaluating the presence of dysfunctional cognitions about moods. Discuss any episodes of medication noncompliance using the medication noncompliance protocol (see Chapter 2).

Homework Review

Review the Treatment Contract and check to see whether treatment team members have signed it. If the patient has not followed through on completing the sections and discussing the contract with treatment team members, engage in problem solving of how to facilitate its completion.

Next, review the patient's assignment of reflecting over previous manic episodes and associated changes in thoughts, feelings, and behaviors. Keep a running list of these either on a dry erase board or on a note pad. This discussion should provide a segue into the content of today's session.

Discussion of Hypomanic Cognitive Errors

Explain to the patient that one of the strategies for preventing relapse is the identification of early warning signs of episodes. The following dialogue can be used to transition to a discussion of hypomanic cognitive errors:

In previous sessions, we've talked a lot about the warning signs of depression and the types of negative thinking biases that can occur in depression. We've discussed the way in which thoughts, feelings, and behaviors are tightly interconnected, for example, the way that you think about something affects both your moods and your behaviors. What I would like to cover today is the detection and prevention of manic episodes. During any of your previous manic or hypomanic episodes, have you noticed that your thinking becomes hyperpositive?

Use probing questions to encourage a discussion of hyperpositive thinking biases. It is also important to note that the hypomanic patient's thinking may be skewed in an irritable way (e.g., misinterpreting innocuous cues for aggressive behavior.)

Facilitate a discussion of the types of thoughts associated with hypomania. Depending upon level of insight and experience with the disorder, patients may vary tremendously in their ability to recall specific cognitive changes. Therefore, it is helpful to direct the patient to the list of typical cognitive errors of hypomania that appears in the workbook (see also the same list provided here). This is done in a similar fashion to the Burns' list of depressive cognitive errors.

List of Hypomanic Cognitive Errors

Positive fortune-telling—being overly optimistic about unknown outcomes

Overreliance on luck—e.g., "I can get away with it."

Underestimating risk or danger—e.g., "It will work out one way or another."

Overly positive appraisal of one's talents and abilities—e.g., "I can do no wrong."

Disqualifying the negative/Minimizing problems/Not thinking through the negative consequences—e.g., "I don't have a care in the world."

Overvaluing of immediate gratification—e.g., "I want what I want when I want it."

Suspiciousness or paranoia—e.g., "Everyone is looking at me."

Misinterpreting the intentions of others—e.g., seeing sexual content or innuendo where there is none ("He/she wants me.") or seeing slights or aggressive content where there is none ("They're out to get me.")

Inappropriate use of humor—e.g., "They think I'm funny."

Seeing special connections or heightened religious significance

The following case vignette demonstrates how hypomanic thoughts may be presented.

Case Vignette

T: This list contains typical thinking biases associated with hypomania. The goal will be for you to recognize these types of thoughts and to intervene before to a full-blown episode of mania. Do you follow me so far?

P: Yeah, I think so.

T: Let's go over some of these together. The first one involves what we call "Positive Fortune-Telling" in which a person becomes overly optimistic about unknown outcomes. Can you ever recall a time when you might have had such thoughts?

P: Well, yes. I remember last spring when I was manic; I began to think that my whole life would be perfect, no matter what. So, I made some risky decisions thinking that everything would be great . . . I predicted it!

T: So, your thoughts affected your behaviors?
(Here, the therapist is helping the patient make the connection between thoughts and behaviors.)

P: Yes, absolutely. I took chances that I never would have normally because I was convinced that everything would have a happy ending.

T: Those types of thoughts also seem to relate to the next several cognitive errors of hypomania on this list: "Overrelying on luck" and "Underestimating risk or danger."

P: Yes, that definitely describes the way I was thinking. I made some risky investments, thinking that I would be lucky and amazingly successful.

T: And how were you feeling during that time?

P: It was like being on a euphoric drug. I was on top of the world.

T: So, it sounds like you were thinking about things in an extremely positive way, feeling euphoric, and taking risks that you normally would not have taken?
(Tying together the relationship between thoughts, feelings, and behaviors)

P: Yes, that pretty much sums it up.

T: And then what happened?

P: I crashed big time. I lost a ton of money and really messed up my financial situation.

T: Do you think if you had noticed the early warning signs of mania, you might have been able to prevent some of the negative consequences you experienced?

P: I guess so. It all seemed to happen so quickly, but I do recall that several of my friends had noticed the symptoms before I did those crazy things. I guess if they had been on my Treatment Contract, I may not have followed through on those crazy investments. I may have listened to them.

T: Do you think that you may have been able to challenge some of your hyperpositive thoughts if you had caught them before they progressed to mania?

P: I certainly hope so, but I wasn't really tuned in to watching out for my thoughts back then.

T: Well, yes, it certainly does take some time and practice to learn how to watch out for those types of thoughts. We will be spending more time together working on this over the next several sessions so that you will be ready to catch these thoughts in the future.

Challenging Hyperpositive Thinking

Explain to the patient that the same techniques can be used to examine hyperpositive thinking as are used to challenge depressive cognitions. In order to demonstrate this, work through an example using a Thought Record (see Figure 15.1).

Explain that early detection is crucial. Cognitive restructuring is rarely effective once a person is in a full-blown manic episode. Therefore, the goal is to recognize and test out hyperpositive thoughts before escalating into a full manic episode.

Situation	Emotion	Automatic thought	Evaluation of automatic thought	Re-rate emotion
(Describe the event that led to the unpleasant emotion)	(Specify sad, angry, etc., and rate the emotion from 0% to 100%)	(Write the automatic thought and rate your belief in the thought from 0% to 100%)	(Evaluate the accuracy of the automatic thought)	(Re-rate the emotion And your belief in the thought from 0% to 100%)
Received a promotion at work	Elated 90%	I am so much smarter than the CEO and I need to tell her on Monday morning how she should change the company. Belief in the thought = 90%	My therapist has encouraged me to wait before acting impulsively. I may be smarter than my boss and the CEO, but I should probably not tell them what to do. Maybe I can put together a proposal with some of my ideas. My mood chart reflects that I'm a bit hypomanic right now so maybe I should focus on getting some sleep.	Elated 75% Belief in the thought = 80%—my belief has not decreased that much, but I have a better plan for presenting my ideas at work.
An attractive man smiled at me on the airplane	Excited 90%	He wants me. I should go talk to him. Belief in the thought = 90%	He might think I'm attractive, but it doesn't necessarily mean that he wants me. These types of thoughts have	Excited 70% Belief in the thought = 50%

Figure 15.1

Example of Completed Thought Record (responses to hypomanic or irritable thoughts)

			gotten me into trouble in the past. Besides, I'm married and want to stay faithful to my husband. I'm a bit elevated and feeling hypersexual right now.	

Figure 15.1 *continued*

Discussion of Strategies to Prevent Hypomanic or Impulsive Behaviors

Once the patient has a grasp on challenging hyperpositive thinking, discuss strategies to interfere with impulsive and risky behaviors. Review the following list of strategies with the patient. Have the patient follow along using the same list in the workbook. These may be introduced to the patient through a discussion of the consequences of past manic episodes.

List of Strategies to Interfere With Impulsive, Hypomanic Behaviors

■ Avoid major financial decisions such as new purchases or major investments. This is done to protect your financial security, so that your long-term financial health is not challenged by the consequences of *overconfidence* from mania. If you feel like you must make a decision when you are feeling positive or high, it is best to check with at least two valued advisors to help you decide whether the decision is sound. This is called the two-person feedback rule. Because a hypomanic mood may lead you to believe that you are thinking faster and better than those around you, it is crucial that you do not discount the advice from these valued advisors.

■ Avoid alcohol and drug use when hypomanic. When hypomanic, you may feel like you can handle alcohol or drug use; it is crucial at these times to know that your judgment is impaired by the mood episode. No good can come from mixing alcohol and drug use with hypomania.

- Avoid relationship decisions. When hypomanic, don't give out your phone number, ask out new people, or engage in sexual behavior with new partners.

- Avoid confrontations. Hypomania and mania often brings irritability. When irritability is high, it may well be worth protecting your job or your relationships by taking a day off work or agreeing with you family members to not have major discussions ("I am really irritable these days from my mood, let's put off any major discussions until I feel better. And if I seem especially caught up on minor issues, know that these issues may be much more manageable for me when my mood normalizes.").

- Avoid using a credit card when hypomanic. When mood episodes strike, you may want to turn over any credit cards with high spending limits to a valued other so that you cannot create substantial debt for yourself during the episode.

Case Vignette

T: So, you were telling me about the negative financial situation that arose due to your risky investments while manic. Has this consequence caused many problems for you?

P: Absolutely! I am still paying for those mistakes. What really kills me is that I had a pretty solid financial situation before that, and now I am barely keeping my head above water.

T: So, it really sounds like you have suffered greatly due to those decisions. How about we talk about some ways to prevent those types of impulsive decisions in the future?

P: Sure.

T: Well, one strategy that can be useful is what we call the "Two-Person Feedback Rule." By using this strategy, you agree to check out any new plans or ideas with two trusted friends or colleagues before taking action. If either of your "advisors" feels that your plan might not be a good idea, then you agree to postpone action for 2 weeks, and reevaluate the plan with your two advisors at that point.

P: Does that sound like something you would be willing to try?

T: Yes. I suppose if I had had that type of strategy in place last year, I may not have followed through on those investments.

P: Do you think that you would have listened to your "advisors?"

T: Maybe I would not have then, but in the future I am willing to make it a policy. I don't want to experience that type of destruction again.

P: Good, I think that is a very wise strategy. After all, most important people in the world who make major decisions have their advisors. For example, the president has his cabinet. Who do you think you might include on yours?

T: Well, I certainly could include some of the same people who are on my Treatment Contract, like my brother and my best friend. When considering business decisions, I may also want to include my colleague, Mike. He's very savvy about these types of decisions and I trust his judgment.

P: Great, it sounds like you are well on your way toward forming a strong cabinet of advisors.

Implementation Problems

The main obstacles in having patients follow through on the aforementioned strategies include a lack of acceptance of bipolar disorder or a yearning for previous manic highs. This is more commonly seen in younger patients, who may not yet have suffered major consequences from manic behaviors. Such patients may be less likely to buy into the fact that manic episodes can be dangerous. Psychoeducational materials can be useful in providing this message in a convincing way. Kay Jamison's book *An Unquiet Mind* can be useful in educating the patient about the dangerous consequences of manic behavior (Jamison, 1997).

If you detect patient yearnings for past manic highs, this certainly should be a top priority for future sessions.

Session Summary

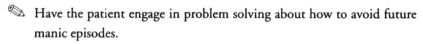

Take a few minutes to review with the patient the most salient points of today's session. It is helpful to consolidate the information and make sure that the patient understands and remembers the important points.

Homework

✎ Have the patient engage in problem solving about how to avoid future manic episodes.

✎ Have the patient finalize the Treatment Contract (if not yet completed).

Treatment Phase 3

In the third phase of treatment, you will continue to emphasize the core tools for change. These tools include cognitive restructuring, problem solving, and activity assignments, as well as in-session rehearsal of all skills to be applied. In this phase of treatment, these skills may be applied to any of a wide range of disorders, symptoms, or life problems.

Format of the Problem-List Phase

Patient care in this phase of treatment is guided not by the session-by-session format used in the first two phases of treatment, but by Case Conceptualization Worksheets that help you decide which problems deserve the most attention in upcoming sessions. However, in all cases, treatment follows the basic format utilized in previous sessions. Each session is formulated into a problem-solving format that includes:

(a) review of the previous week's progress and difficulties

(b) formulation of an agenda for the session and completion of the agenda with attention to in-session rehearsal of concepts

(c) summary of the session content

(d) assignment of homework

This format maintains a consistent focus on the step-by-step, goal-oriented, skill-acquisition approach that is at the heart of this treatment.

Consistent with recent recommendations in the literature, the problem-list phase of treatment is module based. Only patients having select difficulties will receive select interventions. Targets during this phase of treatment are "instrumental" outcomes. Instrumental outcomes, as defined by Rosen and Proctor (1981), are the outcomes therapists wish to manipulate in treatment to achieve ultimate outcomes such as the resolution of depression. For example, Nezu & Nezu's (1993) list of instrumental outcomes for the treatment of depression include the following:

- Increasing pleasant activities

- Decreasing unpleasant activities

- Increase expectations of positive outcomes

- Improving problem-solving abilities

- Increasing communication skills and assertion

- Improving marital and other interpersonal relationships

- Decreasing unrealistic expectations

- Increasing self-reinforcement

- Decreasing negative self-evaluations

- Correcting cognitive distortions

In the current stage of treatment emphasis is placed on a three hierarchical goals:

1. Adequate acquisition of cognitive-behavioral skills emphasized to date

2. Remission of depression

3. Treatment of other life problems

The second goal is presumed to be dependent on the first, and likewise the third goal is presumed to be of secondary importance to depression relief. Nonetheless, the purpose of the Case Conceptualization Worksheets is to direct the therapist to the most relevant instrumental goals for each patient.

Number and Timing of Sessions

The problem-list phase of treatment is designed to last for a maximum of 13 sessions, with the introduction of the final phase of therapy, a well-being focus, by Session 27. However, if the patient is doing well, the principles of well-being therapy can be introduced as early as Session 23 to complement the focus on improving the enjoyment of life that is part of the problem-list phase.

Case Conceptualization Worksheets

The Case Conceptualization Worksheets are for independent use by the therapist to guide the selection of the most appropriate targets for treatment within the constraints of the interventions listed in this protocol. The worksheets are to be used approximately monthly as a way to formalize the therapist's conceptualization of the case and relevant interventions. The worksheets are not designed to be shared with the patient; instead they are used for case conceptualization and planning of interventions only.

The worksheets (1 and 2) are designed to place emphasis first on the full acquisition of the most relevant treatment skills and second, on the application of these skills to additional problem areas.

Case Conceptualization Worksheet 1: Acquisition of Skills Already Presented

The purpose of this worksheet is to help you evaluate the degree to which the patient has learned some of the core skills utilized in treatment. As treatment progresses, the patient will be required to repeatedly call upon these skills as they are applied to new instrumental goals. Accordingly, one of the first goals of the problem-list treatment phase is to help ensure that basic skills have been acquired. If you judge skills to be inadequate, you should apply the corresponding interventions.

This worksheet is *not* to be reviewed in session; instead it is to be reviewed by you when planning future session content. Moreover, the interventions listed below represent the minimum range of interventions that should be considered when deficit areas are observed. If the patient is experiencing multiple skill deficits, you should prioritize which skills are most relevant to the patient's current needs.

Therapeutic Attitude

Has the patient learned an empathetic attitude toward herself or himself with an orientation toward stepwise problem solving? Elements of this skill include the following:

_____ Able to recognize when one is hurt by symptoms or problems and to be oriented toward self-care rather than criticism

_____ Able to inhibit self-criticism and examine useful responses to negative affect

_____ Oriented toward learning new skills and aware of the potential benefits of new skills

_____ Aware of depression as a syndrome, including thought biases and the source of somatic symptoms, disruptions of activity levels and energy, etc.

_____ Aware of bipolar disorder as a disorder, including the need for the acquisition of specific skills to reduce the risk of relapse

_____ Able to apply skills learned in session to problem areas

If "No" to any of the above, consider the following:

Interventions for Therapeutic Attitude

1. Review the model of the disorder (e.g., Session 1, information in the workbook).

2. Review the model of "two therapists" on the case (Session 1).

3. Assign self-monitoring (Thought Record) of the effects of self-criticism.

4. Reemphasize adaptive coaching (Coach B).

5. Examine core beliefs surrounding perfection and self-punishment.

6. Complete Socratic questioning of the effects of self-criticism and other alternatives for responding to negative affect.

7. Role-play the therapeutic attitude by asking the patient to adopt the "therapist" role while you adopt a self-critical perspective.

8. Write out common self-criticisms on an index card, review in session, and rehearse more adaptive alternatives to these statements.

9. Target self-monitoring assignments (Thought Records) to the patient's responses to negative affect.

10. Complete therapeutic problem solving (as per the basic session structure), and then abstract for the patient what was done during the session (i.e., that you responded to the patient with empathy and problem solving).

11. Assess distress tolerance skills; if needed, apply skills from Chapter 22 (Extreme Emotions Module).

Some of the more common targets of cognitive restructuring include the patient's conceptualization of events (particularly social or performance events), the patient's evaluation of his or her own performance, and ongoing evaluation and modification of core beliefs. In these domains, be particularly sensitive to themes of presumed rejection by others, and failure-focused attention (noticing what is not proceeding well) combined with perfectionistic or overly rigid self-standards. In addition to this sensitivity, ensure that component parts of self-monitoring and cognitive restructuring are being applied. The following checklist should be used to assess the adequacy by which the patient has adopted basic cognitive restructuring skills. Problem solving is included as a cognitive restructuring skill that the patient should be applying in daily life.

_____ Able to identify affect
If no, rehearse identification of affect in the session, focusing on the description of emotion in response to events from the patient's week. Discuss the _likely_ emotional responses to these events.

_____ Able to identify automatic thoughts (after the fact)
If no, try to capture automatic thoughts in response to situations described in session.

_____ Able to identify automatic thoughts as they occur
If no, continue with restructuring assignments, asking the patient to "cognitively stop and evaluate" her or his thoughts as soon as a negative emotion is noticed. Alternatively, consider the use of cues for self-monitoring of thoughts (see info on the use of reminder dots in Chapter 2).

_____ Able to generate alternative thoughts
If no, continue to practice cognitive restructuring in the session, with specific assignment of regular rehearsals and monitoring of adaptive (e.g., Coach B metaphor from Session 2) thoughts in response to negative events.

_____ Able to feel a shift in affect from cognitive restructuring
If no, examine the "tone" of cognitive restructuring as well as the accuracy of the alternative thoughts the patient is using. Examine core beliefs around the way a person should treat herself/himself.

_____ Able to recognize habitual negative thoughts
If no, spend session time discussing themes evident in the self-monitoring. Discuss thoughts as being habitual. Assign "capturing" of negative habits during the next week's self-monitoring.

_____ Able to apply problem-solving techniques out of the session

If no, consider the following interventions:

1. Greater modeling of problem solving in session, with fading (reductions) in the therapist's activity level over time (see Chapter 17).

2. Formal assignment of the Problem-Solving Worksheet weekly.

3. Assessment of negative or catastrophic thoughts (e.g., "Why bother? It won't work out anyway"; "Nothing feels better so why try?") that may derail problem solving efforts, followed by restructuring of these thoughts.

4. Role-playing of problem situation to assess or refine skills/alternatives for coping with the situation.

5. Rehearsal (role-play) of solutions to a problem situation, then assignment of its completion during the week, with review of progress the next session.

Activity Assignments

Activity assignments provide a format for the "doing" component of CBT. The goal of activity assignments is to structure life events and activities that best provide a buffer from negative mood states and that directly contribute to a stable, positive affect. In the upcoming phase of treatment, much more attention is devoted to the acquisition of skills to aid the successful completion of activity assignments.

_____ Sufficient buffering events during the week to allow breaks from ongoing stressors (including breaks from boredom)
If no, see Chapter 4.

_____ Regular pleasurable events occur
If no, reapply interventions from Chapters 4 or 5.

_____ Regular mastery/achievement events occur
If no, reapply interventions from Chapters 6 or 7.

_____ Moments of pleasure occur in response to positive events

If no, apply one of the following:

1. Monitor, examine, and restructure cognitions occurring before, during, or after the event.

2. Examine elements of the event, searching for specific moments of loss of pleasure. Reevaluate the target behavior in response to enjoyed or disliked elements of the event.

3. Examine setting conditions influencing the event (e.g., inadequate sleep, worries, and alternative motivations).

4. Examine the skills needed to enjoy the event (e.g., social skills). Provide role-play of the event to allow for a clear assessment and to help skills develop. Consider interventions from Chapter 18 (Social Skills Training Module).

5. Examine the influence of comorbid conditions. Does anxiety interfere with enjoyment? Consider interventions from Chapters 19–22 (Anxiety Management, Breathing and Relaxation Strategies, Anger Management, and Extreme Emotions Modules).

6. Examine core cognitions regarding the "purpose of life" (i.e., the importance or worth of pursuing activities for enjoyment; see Chapter 23).

7. Help the patient develop alternative activities that may lead to more pleasure. Stepwise goal attainment may need to be reviewed.

_____ Patient attends to positive events once completed
If no, complete cognitive restructuring around an appropriate or adaptive attentional focus. Consider assigning self-monitoring of pleasant events (see the Well-Being Module; Chapter 23).

_____ Activity schedule is manageable given the constraints of bipolar disorder.
If no, provide interventions from Chapter 2.

_____ Aversive events occur at a low frequency
If no, complete problem solving or, if the aversive event is in the social realm, assertiveness training (see Chapters 17 and 18).

_____ Patient is able to enjoy unstructured time
If no, consider relaxation training (Chapter 20) or "Worry Time" interventions (Chapter 19). Alternatively, consider a didactic discussion of the use of unstructured time, with review of the way people known to the patient or the therapist may utilize this time. Consider assignment of "trying their skill."

Case Conceptualization Worksheet 2: Additional Targets for Treatment

This worksheet can be used either to troubleshoot potential reasons for nonresponse to interventions for depression or to select targets for treatment as part of relapse-prevention efforts. Relapse-prevention efforts provide the patient with an opportunity to hone cognitive-behavioral skills while reducing risk factors for relapse. This list should be reviewed monthly during the problem-list phase of treatment.

Again, this worksheet is not to be reviewed in session; instead it is to be reviewed by you when planning future session content. If the patient is experiencing multiple skill deficits, you should prioritize which skills are most relevant to the patient's current needs. The suggestions for each problem area represent the minimum set of interventions that should be considered. In many cases, these suggestions refer to subsequent chapters where the interventions are exemplified.

_____ Patient is noncompliant with medication regimen

- Assess noncompliance in a problem-solving format, examining the patient's cognitions regarding medications and their side effects and benefits (see Chapter 2).

- If needed, role-play the discussions the patient may want to have with her or his prescribing physician.

- For problems of irregular medication use unrelated to motivation deficits, utilize cue-control procedures to cue medication use, and review compliance information in Chapter 2.

- For problems of irregular medication use because of concerns around weight gain, apply monitoring of food or caloric intake and problem-solving interventions (including increasing activities and exercise). However, weight loss is not a central focus of the treatment. If major problems with obesity, anorexia nervosa, or bulimia exist, alternative treatment may need to be considered.

_____ Patient reports irregular sleep or sleep disruption

- Apply sleep hygiene procedures, with monitoring of outcome.

_____ Substance use is of concern

- Assess degree of substance use in a problem-solving format, examining the patient's cognitions regarding substance use, and discuss the risks of such use. Identify cues for substance use, and rehearse alternative behaviors to those cues.

- If the patient meets criteria for substance abuse or dependence, refer the patient to a substance use counselor (as per Pathway recommendations) and continue with CBT focusing on mood and other relapse-prevention issues.

_____ Anxiety interferes with activity goals or pleasant events

- Utilize cognitive restructuring interventions to examine probability overestimations and catastrophization (see Chapter 19—Anxiety Management Module).

- Evaluate the role of worry, and consider assigning worry times (see Chapter 19).

- Introduce relaxation skills if relevant (see Chapter 20).

_____ Avoidance interferes with activity goals or pleasant events.

- Conduct self-monitoring and cognitive restructuring around feared events.

- Introduce stepwise exposure with attention to disconfirmation of fears (see Chapter 19).

_____ Interpersonal relationships are not satisfying.

- Examine the role of loneliness as a contributing symptom to depression.

- Conduct problem solving of other venues for social activities, and assign these activities in a step-wise fashion.

- Examine dysfunctional cognitions that may make interpersonal interactions more threatening.

- Examine social skills (e.g., using role-play rehearsals); if necessary, teach assertiveness (see Chapter 18).

- Discuss active listening and communication skills. Assign home practice and role-play alternatives (see Chapter 18).

_____ Aversive interpersonal events contribute to symptoms

- Complete problem-solving focusing on ways to reduce these events (see Chapter 17).

- Investigate the role of assertiveness in helping the patient reduce socially aversive events (if needed, apply interventions from Chapter 18).

- Plan in additional buffering or pleasant events (see Chapter 2).

_____ Repeated emotional crises interfere with application of skills

- Teach distress tolerance as a buffering skill until problem solving and cognitive restructuring alternatives can be rehearsed (see Chapter 22).

_____ Patient's goals are not adequately achieved:

- Review stepwise goal attainment in a problem-solving format (see Chapter 17)

- Discuss modification of goals if limiting life circumstances preclude goal attainment at this time.

Chapter 17 | *Problem-Solving Module*

(Corresponds to chapter 11 of the workbook)

Materials Needed

■ Problem-Solving Worksheet

Outline

■ Set agenda (as in previous sessions)

■ Review Mood Chart (as in previous sessions)

■ Review homework (as in previous sessions)

■ Introduce problem solving

■ Review the steps of problem solving

■ Introduce the Problem-Solving Worksheet

■ Summarize session (as in previous sessions)

■ Assign homework (as in previous sessions)

Introduction to Problem Solving

As discussed previously, depressed patients often have a limited view of the world and engage in narrow thinking patterns that can be problematic. Many depressed patients approach problem solving in much the same way. That is, there is a tendency to view problems as unsolvable or to have limited conceptualizations about solutions. Problem-solving considers all solutions as viable until they are evaluated more closely. The use of problem solving does not guarantee a perfect solution, but does ensure that the patient considers the problems and solutions more thoroughly before making decisions or "giving up."

Steps to Problem Solving

Components of a traditional problem solving approach include the following:

1. Identifying the problem

2. Clearly defining the problem (what about the situation makes it bothersome?)

3. Brainstorming a list of all possible solutions, even those that may seem silly or impossible

4. Evaluating the solutions (advantages and disadvantages of each)

5. Selecting a solution or combination of solutions (taking into account the benefits and liabilities of each solution)

6. Implementing the solution

7. Evaluating the effectiveness of the solution

The goal of this intervention is to teach the overall problem-solving approach to patients, yet encourage the use of individual steps in a less formal manner to address daily problems. The use of individual components of a problem-solving strategy can be modeled in session. In addition, patients may need help in challenging irrational thinking that accompanies and/or impedes effective problem solving.

The following case vignette provides an example of how to teach a patient the problem-solving technique.

P: I am not sure what to do. I am not going to pass the course I am taking. It's only 4 weeks into the semester and I already have a D. There's no hope! I should have known better, given that in the last course I took I got a C-.

T: What is it about this situation that is problematic for you?

P: Well, I can't get a D in this class or I will not be able to matriculate into my major. But, if I drop the class and wait to take it the next time it is offered, then I will be behind a whole year. Like I said; I have no idea what to do. I guess I wasn't cut out for college in the first place.

T: Now that I understand your problem, let's consider options for what to do about it.
Initially, the therapist may take a more active role in suggesting solutions and fading out suggestions as the patient improves her ability to generate solutions.

P: I told you my options. Either, I drop the class, or I fail it!
Therapist lists these options on the Problem-Solving Worksheet and then suggests some more (a copy of the worksheet for your use is provided in the apppendix along with a sample completed copy to use as a model).

T: Would you be open to some other suggestions?

P: Of course.

T: What are some things that you can do that may help to improve your grade?

P: If I knew I would be doing them.

T: Okay. How about getting involved in a study group with classmates?

P: I guess that is an option.
Therapist adds study group to the list of options on the Problem-Solving Worksheet (see appendix).

T: And what about talking to the professor to see if she has any suggestions for improving your grade?

P: She is not very approachable. But I could give it a shot. Oh yeah, she did announce last class that there was a TA who could tutor those of us who are having a hard time. I didn't write down his name because I figured he probably couldn't help me anyway. But, maybe I will try that.

When helping a patient problem solve, you should assist the patient in developing a list of alternative solutions. Discourage evaluation of solutions until the next step and reiterate the notion of brainstorming ideas. As the patient pursues solutions, her sense of hopelessness may decrease and an affective shift may occur. After each step in the problem-solving process, revisit and challenge the original distorted thoughts with the patient.

T: It seems to me that we have been able to come up with a number of alternative solutions in addition to dropping or failing the class.

P: I guess we have. I really didn't think about these options before.

T: In light of these new options, do you feel and/or think any differently about the situation?

P: I feel much better about the situation. I think there may be a way for me to pass this course after all.

It may not be necessary to carry out all steps of the problem-solving strategy with every patient. For example, if the patient has experienced an affective shift and is more open to alternatives, it may not be necessary to assist her in formally carrying out final steps of problem solving. Rather, at this point you may want to briefly discuss what the patient will do to finish problem solving for this particular situation, and then move on. It is important to include this topic in the agenda for the next session to see how the problem was resolved. On the other hand, if the patient remains hopeless about the situation, it may be advisable to continue a more formal approach to problem solving. If this is the course, the next step is to evaluate the list of solutions by examining the advantages and disadvantages of each solution.

T: Now that we have this list of potential solutions, let's rate each one of them.

P: I can tell you now which one is probably the best to do.

T: Hold off on trying to make a decision for now. Wait until you rate the good and bad aspects of each proposed solution. Let's start by having you identify what is good and bad about each solution. (For each solution, have the patient clearly identify the pros and cons, making a written list for each.)

T: Given this evaluation, which solution seems best? (Guide patient through this process.)

If the patient continues to have difficulty, more time and/or information may be necessary to solve the problem. Help the patient determine what she can do to gather more information and revisit the problem during a future session. If the patient does adopt a solution or a combination of solutions, the next step is to formulate a plan for carrying out the solution. Again, some patients can do this with very little guidance.

The final step of problem solving is to evaluate the effectiveness of the plan. This is conducted in a subsequent session based on the specifics of the plan. Regardless of which formal steps are addressed in session, it is recommended that this final step be covered to ensure follow-through and discussion of the outcome of problem solving.

Chapter 18 *Social Skills Training Module*

(Corresponds to chapter 12 of the workbook)

Materials Needed

- Hierarchy of Social Situations

Outline

- Set agenda (as in previous sessions)

- Review Mood Chart (as in previous sessions)

- Review homework (as in previous sessions)

- Introduce social skills training

- Address general social skills

- Address assertiveness

- Summarize session (as in previous sessions)

- Assign homework (as in previous sessions)

Introduction to Social Skills Training

Patients with bipolar disorder may experience difficulties with social situations for a number of reasons. In some cases, comorbid social anxiety may inhibit their social interactions and increase difficulties in situations requiring assertiveness or conflict management skills. For other patients, social skills deficits may stem from their mood state, so that they experience frequent conflict with others when irritable or depressed, or violate social norms when they become hypomanic. Careful evaluation of the nature of the patient's social difficulties is required to tailor this module to patients' needs. Two different social skills are presented in this module. The first section addresses more global skills required in social interactions, including verbal and nonverbal communication skills. The second section of the module focuses on assertiveness and conflict resolution skills.

Patients may benefit from some or all of the skills presented; the extent of the training will depend on the nature of the skills deficit, and agreement between you and the patient regarding goals of treatment. Regardless of the specific behavioral skills deficits evinced by the patient, you should carefully monitor the presence of any cognitive distortions in social situations. For example, patients may have a number of negative cognitions regarding interpersonal rejection or may have unrealistic expectations about their performance in social situations. In this case, cognitive restructuring will be an essential adjunct to a behavioral social skills approach.

General Social Skills Training

This section is designed to address the verbal and nonverbal skills involved in effectively initiating or maintaining interpersonal interactions. In addition to verbal skills, behaviors include positive social interaction skills such as smiling, laughing, and making appropriate eye contact.

Social Skill Assessment

Assessment includes an overview of behavioral strengths as well as weaknesses. If the patient is unable to articulate specific areas of difficulty, you can ask him to imagine himself in various social situations and report his feelings, thoughts, and behaviors. This may provide clues about any cognitive distortions in social situations, as well as specific behavioral difficulties. Likewise, review of situations in which the patient previously experienced difficulty may yield targets for treatment. In social skills training, you should set specific behavioral goals with the patient. Care should be taken to ensure that these goals are both realistic and focused on behaviors rather than feeling states (for example, "I will talk to one person at the party" rather than, "I will go to the party and not feel nervous").

Strategies for Social Skills Training

Once these goals have been established, social skills training involves a combination of strategies:

1. modeling of social behaviors

2. coaching or instructional training

3. behavioral rehearsal

4. corrective feedback

5. reinforcement of social skills

In the first phase of social skills training, describe and discuss the desired behavior with the patient. Identify specific difficulties in implementing the behavior. Cognitive restructuring is a useful adjunct to social skills training, in that difficulties with social behaviors are often accompanied by distorted expectations about social behavior and negative cognitions regarding performance in social situations.

Ensure that the patient is aware of expected behaviors and the context in which the behavior may be appropriately (versus inappropriately) displayed. For example, coworkers at the office, close friends at a party, or strangers on the subway may perceive sharing personal information very differently. Discuss specific examples of how the same skill will be adapted for use in different situations. Also model appropriate use of the skills.

Situation	Level of Difficulty (0–100)
Saying "hello" to a stranger	20
Walking into a crowded restaurant	35
Initiating a conversation with a coworker	50
Initiating a conversation with a group of three coworkers	70
Asking a coworker for help with a project	95

Figure 18.1

Example of Completed Hierarchy of Social Situations

Hierarchy of Social Situations

As part of the first phase of skills training, work with the patient to devise a hierarchy of social situations (from least difficult to most difficult), which will inform graduated exposure tasks later in treatment. A blank Hierarchy of Social Situations for the patient's use can be found in the workbook. A sample hierarchy is shown in Figure 18.1.

Using behavioral rehearsal, the patient is provided with the opportunity to practice the skills learned in session. At first, this is done using role-plays. As the patient becomes more comfortable implementing the skills, encourage him to practice the skills both in session through in-vivo exposure tasks and on his own using home practice assignments. These tasks are graduated, meaning that they increase in difficulty as the patient masters the skills. The hierarchy is a useful tool for structuring these tasks and assignments. To enhance compliance with home practice, you should ensure that the goals for the home practice are clearly defined, and that potential difficulties are discussed in session (see the following case vignette).

Case Vignette

T: It will take a little more time before you become comfortable with some of these new skills. Remember, any new behavior will feel awkward at first, but as you use it more and more, it will start to become more routine. It's a little bit like riding a bicycle or learning to play a new sport. What we have to think about are ways that you can continue to practice this skill outside of the session. Do you have any ideas about what kind of home practice you would like to do this week?

P: I could ask my friend Roger to go to a movie. I haven't seen him in a while.

T: Okay. Do you have a sense of when you would ask him?

P: Well, if we go see a movie, it would have to be on Saturday, so I guess I'll call and ask him by Thursday night.

T: Do you have a sense of what you'll say to Roger, or is that something that you would like to plan here?

P: No, I think I know what I'll say. I'll do the same thing that we practiced before.

T: Sounds good. I'm wondering how hard this will be for you to do.

P: It should be okay, because I'm already pretty friendly with Roger. Maybe a 35 on the difficulty scale.

T: That sounds reasonable. Is there anything that could happen that would make this more difficult for you to do?

P: Well, definitely if he says no. That would be terrible!

T: Let's spend a little time talking about this, because it seems as though it could be really tough for you if Roger refuses.

Behavioral Experiments

If the patient has expressed a number of distorted thinking patterns about social interactions, behavioral experiments may be integrated into the sessions. Behavioral experiments enable the patient to disconfirm beliefs using direct behavioral evidence. Encourage the patient to set up "experiments" in which his belief is designated as one hypothesis, and a competing (more realistic) belief is designated as a second hypothesis. Ask the patient to carefully observe the outcome of the experiment and analyze the evidence for and against each hypothesis.

Corrective feedback is particularly important in social skills training to enable the patient to modify his behavior. Traditionally, the behavioral practice is critiqued by the therapist (and in some cases, other participants in the practice). This critique should incorporate positive feedback—pointing out which aspects of the behavioral practice were completed successfully, as well as constructive feedback about areas for improvement. Clearly, this feedback must be provided in a sensitive manner, and only within a supportive context. You should also obtain the patient's own impressions about his performance. Examine significant discrepancies between the patient and your impressions; these may warrant cognitive restructuring. Provide additional behavioral practice and feedback until the patient feels that he has mastered the skill. Additional reinforcement and praise for appropriate social skills is important, both to enhance the application of the skills and to maintain rapport (see following case vignette).

Case Vignette

T: You did a great job with this practice. I noticed that you were really able to make good eye contact and spoke in a clear tone of voice. Does that fit with your impressions?

P: I guess so. I felt so nervous, but I was trying really hard to remember what we had talked about with the eye-contact business.

T: Yeah, and even though you were nervous, you were really able to do it. Is there anything else that you thought you handled well during the practice?

P: Let me think. Well, I met my goal of asking the other person three questions.

T: That's true. Overall, how do you think you did during the practice?

P: Pretty well!

T: Is there anything that you think you could use a little more work with?

P: Definitely answering questions in a conversation. I find it really hard to not just give yes or no answers—I'd really like to say more, but I just can't.

Incorporating Strategies for Other Behaviors

Although not a central focus of social skills training, strategies to manage other behaviors that interfere with social relations may be incorporated into this treatment module. For example, aggressive behaviors, emotional dysregulation, and irritability may negatively impact the patient's ability to implement the skills learned in session. In this case, it is appropriate to incorporate treatment strategies targeting these other areas of difficulty within a social-skills training approach. Finally, social isolation may be a significant problem for a number of patients with bipolar disorder. Consequently, strategizing around increasing social interactions will be an important target of treatment. For example, the patient may become involved in community groups, activities, or interest groups in his area. If the social skills learned in treatment are to be maintained, the patient must have the opportunity to practice these social skills on a regular basis.

Assertiveness Training

Even if the more general social skills module is selected, it is not necessary to spend time conducting a full tutorial on assertion training with every patient. Rather, assess the level of skill the patient already has, and adapt training to meet his individual needs. For example, many patients have a reasonable level of assertion skills, but have difficulty using them because of faulty cognitions about their ability to use these skills or what others may think of them.

One strategy for assessing patient's level of assertiveness skills is to have the patient present a social situation in which unassertive behavior may have occurred. Gather information about the situation and give the patient an opportunity to demonstrate what would have been considered assertive behavior. (See following case vignette.)

Case Vignette

P: It was terrible! I waited in the hallway for over an hour to talk with my boss and she just walked by. I really needed her direction to complete the project I am working on.

T: Why were you waiting in the hall so long?

P: Well, she was meeting with a couple of coworkers and then her phone rang and then who knows what she was doing after that.

T: If she was in her office and you wanted to talk with her, why were you waiting in the hallway?

P: I was nervous. I wasn't sure what to say to her. I didn't want her to think I was stupid or slacking on the job.

T: OK. Let's assume you could be assured that she would not think you were stupid or slacking on the job, how would you have handled the situation? *(Here the therapist is trying to assess for faulty cognitions to see if skill deficit is more likely leading to difficulty being assertive.)*

P: Who knows? I am so bad at asking for help. I plan on going in for help and walk out not getting the help I need. In fact, I usually walk out with her giving me even more work when I go in to ask for help.

However, if the following discussion occurs under the same circumstances, it may suggest that skill level is sufficient, but that faulty cognitions may account for lack of assertiveness:

T: Okay. Let's assume you could be assured that she would not think you were stupid or slacking on the job, how would you have handled the situation? *(Here again the therapist is trying to assess for faulty cognitions to see if skill deficit is more likely leading to difficulty being assertive.)*

P: Well, I would not have waited so long in the hallway, and I would have knocked on the door.

T: And what might have you said to her?

P: I would say: "I am glad I caught you. I could really use your help by bouncing some ideas off of you and getting feedback." But, she probably would ask me to come back later because she is always so busy.

T: If she did ask you to come back, what would you have done?

P: I would have asked to set up a specific time to meet and get my questions answered. She usually responds well to setting up a time. But even then, I would still feel really stupid. I mean I should be able to do this stuff on my own. They hired me to do it and I am just so tense that I never get it on my own. I don't know if I even deserve this job. Why did they hire me in the first place?

Both examples deserve additional information gathering, using the same strategy. If skill deficit demonstrates itself as in the first example, more traditional assertion training is warranted. If lack of assertion appears to be related more to faulty cognitions (as was the case in the second example), then application of cognitive therapy strategies to address thoughts in these social situations may prove more beneficial to enhance assertiveness.

Identifying Assertive, Aggressive, and Passive Behaviors

In some cases, the patient may benefit from more extensive assertiveness training. Initial treatment goals are to clarify and differentiate assertive from passive or aggressive behaviors. Explain that the problem with nonassertive behaviors is that they tend to increase stress levels and feelings of frustration. Passive behaviors may allow for resentment to build up, which can negatively impact relationships. Alternatively, aggressive behaviors may increase conflict with others, and feelings of shame, guilt, or regret. Often, the individual may cycle between these two extremes, alternating between passive and aggressive behaviors.

Passivity can be defined as a way of behaving whereby we pay a great deal of attention to others' needs, rights, and wishes, but minimize or ignore our own. Aggressiveness refers to a pattern of behavior where we demand that our own wishes, needs, and rights be considered while paying little attention to the needs of others. In contrast, assertiveness is a way of behaving that respects our wishes, needs, and rights and those of the other person.

It may be particularly helpful to identify concrete examples of these modes of communication. If the patient experiences difficulty generating personally relevant situations, you may present several different scenarios, and together with the patient, come up with passive, aggressive, and assertive responses to the situation. Possible scenarios include the following:

- *Someone asks you for a ride home and it is inconvenient for you because you have several errands to run and the drive will take you out of your way. What can you say?*

- *You would like to ask your boss for a raise. What do you say?*

- *A pushy salesperson is trying to convince you to buy a stereo that is significantly more expensive than you had planned. How do you respond?*

- *You've been waiting for 20 minutes in line at the bank. Suddenly, someone cuts in front of you. What do you say?*

- *The phone rings as you are preparing dinner—it's a good friend of yours. How can you handle the situation?*

- *Your sister asks to borrow money for the second time this month—you have some extra money that you've been putting aside to buy something that you've wanted for a long time. What do you tell her?*

The core of assertion training is teaching the patient differences between assertive, aggressive, and passive behavior. Then, modeling, coaching, and behavioral rehearsal can be employed, providing an opportunity for the patient to practice assertive behavior.

The following case vignette illustrates a patient who believes that being assertive means being aggressive or "mean," and is therefore, passive with friends. In this example, the patient is taught the difference between assertive, aggressive, and passive behavior.

Case Vignette

P: When she calls me and asks me to watch her kids, I just can't say no to her. She calls at least three or four times a week. It is really interfering with me getting my stuff done on those days.

T: So when she asks for your help, you say yes even if you don't want to do it, or it's not convenient for you?

P: Yeah. I get so mad at myself for saying yes, but it is even harder to say no.

T: Have you ever said no?

P: On a couple of occasions. But I lied about why I couldn't do it. I made up some really great excuse so she would believe me.

T: What would happen if you said no and told the truth about why you couldn't do it?

P: That would be cruel. I don't think she would think very highly of me. She would probably think I was a mean person. I would feel really bad. You see, that is why I don't act what you call assertive. I just don't have it in my heart to be mean.

T: I think you may be confusing being assertive with being aggressive. Being assertive doesn't imply that you are mean or that your behavior is malicious in any way. In fact, behaving assertively helps to communicate your true feelings or desires in a thoughtful way that helps both you and the other person to feel understood.

P: So saying no to my friend and making clear what I want isn't aggressive?

T: It doesn't have to be. Sure if you said no and just hung up the phone on your friend or yelled at her for asking again—that could be considered aggressive. On the other hand, if you kindly and firmly decline while taking her feelings and your needs into consideration at the same time, that is considered assertive. Then there is being passive . . . *(Make sure the distinction between the three styles is clear. Provide examples, including the current situation in which the patient was behaving in a passive manner. See if she can identify her behavior as passive in this situation.)*

P: Yeah, well how do I just start being assertive after all these years?

T: Well, that is the next step. I am happy to provide some suggestions, and we can practice your new skills together before you try it out with others. The important thing to remember is that behaving assertively is a skill that takes time, effort, and practice to develop.

Steps to Assertiveness

Effective assertiveness communication entails two basic skills. Initially, the individual must "step back" from the situation and reflect on the course of action to be taken. Secondly, the individual must respond to situational demands in an assertive manner. The first step can itself be broken down into a series of behaviors:

■ Decreasing emotional arousal—taking a step back from the situation to calm down; going for a walk; doing a brief relaxation exercise; deep breathing (or another appropriate calming strategy)

■ Clarifying the nature of the problem. Examining your own feelings and thoughts about the situation.

■ Identifying any distorted patterns of thinking that may be impacting your ability to behave effectively in the situation. Challenging negative, unrealistic, or judgmental thinking patterns.

■ Deciding on which behavior(s) may be appropriate. For example, letting go of the situation versus expressing feelings to the other person.

The second step of assertiveness training focuses on communication skills. Assertive communication entails:

■ Describing the situation to the other person. Reporting the facts as objectively as possible, attempting not to mix in feelings. The reporting should be situation-specific and refer to the current problem at-hand, rather than bringing up a series of past difficulties.

■ Expressing feelings about the situation using "I" statements, as opposed to "You". For example, saying, "I feel upset when . . . " versus, "You messed up when . . . " By taking responsibility for your feelings, you are more likely to engender a positive, nondefensive reaction from others.

■ Asking for what you want in a straightforward, specific manner.

■ Explaining how the suggested change will be beneficial to both parties. Making a positive statement about the other person.

In addition to assertiveness skills, it is important to encourage the patient to identify times when he is most and least able to engage in effective social problem-solving and assertive communication. For example, if the patient is experiencing intense mood symptoms, it may be advisable to postpone discussion of stressful topics until he has recuperated. Family members may be involved in this process by agreeing to limit or delay conflicts or disagreements until the patient is in a more stable mood state.

In addition, encourage family members and the patient to identify signs that discussions are becoming overly distressing, and to mutually set limits on the intensity of discussions. You can problem solve with the patient alternative behaviors that can be applied during family conflict situations, such as taking "time-out" from a heated debate until cooler heads can prevail.

Chapter 19 | *Management of Comorbid Anxiety Disorders Module*

Therapist Note

■ *This module is necessary only if comorbid anxiety disorders are present.* ■

Optional Materials Needed

- ■ *Mastery of Your Anxiety and Panic, Fourth Edition* (Craske & Barlow, 2006)

- ■ *Mastery of Your Anxiety and Worry, Second Edition* (Zinbarg, Craske, & Barlow, 2006)

- ■ *Mastery of Obsessive Compulsive Disorder* (Foa & Kozak, 2004).

Outline

- ■ Set agenda (as in previous sessions)

- ■ Review Mood Chart (as in previous sessions)

- ■ Review homework (as in previous sessions)

- ■ Assess comorbid anxiety disorders

- ■ Target symptoms of obsessive-compulsive disorder if present

- ■ Target symptoms of panic disorder if present

- ■ Target symptoms of general anxiety disorder if present

- Summarize session (as in previous sessions)

- Assign homework (as in previous sessions)

Comorbid Anxiety Disorders

Anxiety disorders such as obsessive-compulsive disorder and panic disorder frequently co-occur with bipolar mood disorders. For example, a current comorbid diagnosis of panic disorder is found in greater than 20% of patients with bipolar disorder. Such anxiety disorders can hinder the effectiveness of the treatment interventions included in this guide. For example, a depressed bipolar patient who has comorbid panic disorder with agoraphobia is unlikely to implement a schedule of pleasurable activities designed to enhance her enjoyment of life. Likewise, a patient who is plagued by obsessive thoughts of contamination may be unable to engage in productive problem solving regarding ongoing life difficulties. Therefore, in the context of this protocol, several sessions may be used to target symptoms of comorbid anxiety disorders. This guide will not attempt to summarize the wealth of information on CBT of anxiety disorders. For this reason, three supplemental readings on comorbid conditions are recommended. The first is treatment of panic disorder as guided by the therapist guide for Panic Control Treatment (Craske & Barlow, 2006). The second is treatment of worry and generalized anxiety as guided by the manual *Mastery of Your Anxiety and Worry, Therapist Guide, Second Edition* (Zinbarg et al., 2006), and the third is treatment of obsessions and compulsions as guided by the manual *Mastery of Obsessive-Compulsive Disorder, Therapist Guide* by Foa and Kozak, (2004). The following section will detail the special issues in treating anxiety disorders in patients with bipolar disorder.

Special Issues in the Treatment of Obsessive-Compulsive Disorder (OCD)

The treatment of OCD in bipolar patients presents unique difficulties. Pharmacological agents, such as selective serotonin reuptake inhibitors

(SSRIs), are often quite effective in managing OCD symptoms. However, these medications may trigger mania in bipolar patients. Therefore, cognitive-behavioral interventions play an especially important role in treating comorbid OCD symptoms in bipolar patients. A predictable struggle in treatment arises when the patient's OCD symptoms improve in response to the use of antidepressants, while their symptoms of hypomania worsen. It is often at this point that the therapist must help the patient weigh the pros and cons of future manic episodes versus OCD symptoms.

Many of the techniques included in the coping with mania sections of this guide can be useful in monitoring and challenging such manic symptoms. Typically, the patient must hold some degree of belief in the efficacy of CBT for OCD in order to agree to taper antidepressants. As the patient progresses using exposure and response prevention strategies, she may be more willing to gradually discontinue antidepressant treatment and rely more heavily on the use of cognitive-behavioral strategies to manage OCD symptoms.

The use of "exposure and response prevention" has been the gold standard of cognitive behavioral treatment for OCD. The goal of exposure/response prevention (E/RP) is to enable extinction to anxiety-provoking obsessions and situations by decreasing both passive and active (i.e., ritualizing) avoidance. Treatment begins with a careful assessment of the specific content and frequency of the patient's obsessions and compulsions. Patients are asked to rate the degree of difficulty associated with preventing their compulsive behaviors. Using this information, the therapist and patient construct a hierarchy of exposures ranging from mild to severe difficulty. For example, an OCD patient with contamination fears may experience mild anxiety (e.g., a rating of "10" on a 0–100 scale) when shaking hands with someone without subsequently washing her hands. Early in treatment, he would be assigned to pursue such handshaking exposures. Gradually, he would pursue increasingly difficult exposures, until eventually reaching the most anxiety-provoking exposures on the hierarchy (e.g., using a public restroom with an associated anxiety rating of "100"). For additional information on setting up exposure hierarchies and implementing exposure and response prevention strategies, please see Foa and Kozak (2004).

Also, using Thought Records and cognitive restructuring may be helpful in challenging obsessive blasphemous or unacceptable sexual thoughts. Many OCD patients believe that having these thoughts are as bad as acting on them. Alternatively, some OCD patients may believe that simply thinking about something terrible will cause it to happen (e.g., thinking about their spouse's plane will cause it to crash). Therefore, cognitive restructuring techniques, such as those outlined in the early sessions of this manual, can be used to challenge and test the validity of such obsessional thoughts.

Special Issues in the Treatment of Panic Disorder

As noted previously, panic disorder frequently occurs in patients with bipolar disorder. Often the symptoms of panic are exacerbated as the symptoms of depression worsen. Such a worsening cycle of panic and depression can be paralyzing and can contribute to a patient's sense of being vulnerable, trapped, and hopeless. There is also evidence that co-occurring panic attacks can increase the likelihood of suicide. Therefore, whenever possible, it is essential that the CBT of comorbid panic disorder be included in this protocol. Please refer to *Mastery of Your Anxiety and Panic, Therapist Guide, Fourth Edition* (Craske & Barlow, 2006) for an overview of this approach.

Even if you have limited experience in treating patients with panic disorder, many of the techniques learned in earlier sections of this manual will help to guide treatment. First, educate the patient about the nature of panic disorder and the "fear of fear" cognitive-behavioral model of panic disorder as illustrated in Figure 19.1. Thus, similarly to the treatment of bipolar disorder, the patient must first understand the nature of her panic disorder and the associated role of thoughts, feelings, and behaviors. Use cognitive interventions, similar to those used in previous sessions, to help the patient challenge the cognitive distortions associated with panic attacks.

Relaxation strategies, such as diaphragmatic breathing and progressive muscle relaxation are not core interventions for panic disorder, in part

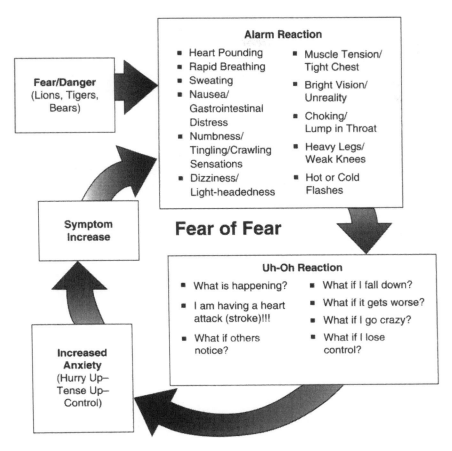

Figure 19.1

Fear-of-Fear Cycle

because some patients may use these techniques as part of a desperate (and anxiogenic) attempt to ward off symptoms. As such, "interoceptive exposure" exercises are the most crucial interventions used in the treatment of panic disorder. Such exercises involve the systematic and controlled elicitation of feared physical sensations that occur during panic attacks. The goal of interoceptive exposure is to help the patient decrease her fear of such bodily sensations (e.g., dizziness and light-headedness). Additionally, in vivo exposures are used to help the patient decrease her agoraphobic avoidance of feared situations. Please refer to the recommended manual for more information on the rationale and conduction of interoceptive exposures.

Many patients with bipolar disorder have numerous, realistic concerns regarding finances, interpersonal difficulties, etc. A small proportion of bipolar patients may also have comorbid generalized anxiety disorder (GAD), in which their anxiety and worry is excessive and difficult to control. For such patients, several strategies can be used to help manage these symptoms. The use of cognitive restructuring to challenge such cognitive distortions (e.g., catastrophizing) can be quite helpful. Relaxation strategies, such as diaphragmatic breathing and progressive muscle relaxation, can be used to help the patient manage the physiological arousal associated with anxious cognitions. Additionally, the problem-solving method as described in Chapter 17 should be used to give the patient tools for managing real-life problems more effectively.

For some patients, the use of prescribed "worry time" can also be helpful. By setting aside specific times during the day to "worry," the patient may be relieved of intrusive worrying throughout the day. These worry times should be scheduled to occur several hours prior to bedtime, and should be conducted at a place for "work" (e.g., at a desk, but not in the family room or bedroom). Patients are to save up worries during the day, and then exclusively focus on these worries during the prescribed time, and to write out the core worries. Writing down the worries will help some patients observe their worries more objectively. Forty-five minutes is allowed for worry; at the end of this time patients may want to apply relaxation skills (see Chapter 20). Then, worries are to be saved up for the next 47 hr until the next worry time. Over the first week of applying this technique, patients begin to report less worry during the day, because of the focusing of worry during a single time. Moreover, patients may complain that their worry time is bothersome because "my worry is a waste of time, I just turn the same thing over and over again in my head." If this occurs, use this cognition to help patients further reduce the habit of worry and substitute in problem solving if needed for actual concerns.

In addition to the worry time intervention, cognitive-restructuring techniques used for depression have excellent application to generalized anxiety. In particular, cognitive-restructuring efforts should attend to anxiogenic thoughts that are based on (1) overestimates of the probability of negative outcomes, and (2) overestimations of the degree of catastrophe of these outcomes should they occur. Helping patients attend to these two distortions during thought monitoring can be effective in reducing anticipatory anxiety and worry. Please refer to *Mastery of Your Anxiety and Worry, Therapist Guide, Second Edition* (Zinbarg et al. 2006) for more information on cognitive-behavioral interventions for GAD.

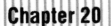

Chapter 20 · *Breathing and Relaxation Strategies Module*

(Corresponds to chapter 13 of the workbook)

Materials Needed

- 8-muscle group progressive muscle relaxation (PMR) script

Outline

- Set agenda (as in previous sessions)

- Review Mood Chart (as in previous sessions)

- Review homework (as in previous sessions)

- Introduce breathing and relaxation skills

- Teach diaphragmatic breathing

- Teach progressive muscle relaxation

- Summarize session (as in previous sessions)

- Assign homework (as in previous sessions)

Introduction to Breathing and Relaxation Skills

Breathing and relaxation skills are among the most generic of psychosocial interventions for anxiety and stress. In short, these techniques are the "aspirin" of CBT: offering some relief for a variety of conditions, but a specific treatment for almost none. Relaxation as a coping procedure can be helpful when the patient is anxious, angry, irritable, or frustrated, though it can be applied during other mood states as well.

In all cases, relaxation and breathing techniques should be taught when the patient is relatively calm, and then applied, with practice, to successively higher-stress situations.

Diaphragmatic Breathing Procedures

Breathing retraining is simply a process of teaching the individual to identify the difference between two ways of filling the lungs. One is to throw the chest outwards and outwards, expanding the chest cavity and bringing in air. The second is to let the chest simply relax, and drop the diaphragm down, again expanding the chest cavity and sucking in air. When the diaphragm pushes upward, air is expelled.

One of the most common strategies for teaching this technique is to have the patient sit with one hand on his chest and the other hand on his abdomen (just above the navel). Model this behavior for the patient. Then, ask the patient to attend to the rise and fall of his hands during breathing, noticing the difference in sensation. By noticing what is done to alternatively make the chest or abdomen move, the patient can learn to breathe more diaphragmatically. During a correct diaphragmatic breath, the abdomen moves outward (during expansion), and then drops back during exhalation. Instruct the patient to feel this movement, but he should not purposefully move the abdominal muscles in and out: it is the diaphragm's movement that causes the stomach to fall outward.

To aid acquisition of diaphragmatic breathing, it is helpful to offer a number of different ways to practice "feeling" each type of breathing. Strategies to better "feel" the diaphragm at work include the following:

1. Have the patient practice laughing with his hand in place. During laughing, the diaphragm tightens, allowing a person to feel tension during each "ho, ho, ho." When breathing in after laughing, the person may spontaneously take a diaphragmatic breath.

2. With hands in place, have the patient slowly expel all air as if he were blowing out an endless series of birthday candles. Rather than inhaling after this exercise, simply instruct the patient to "relax." Immediately upon the relaxation of the candle blowing effort, ask the patient to begin to blow again. Many individuals find that when they relax, they spontaneously refill the lungs with a diaphragmatic breath.

3. Ask the patient to interlace his fingers and place his hands behind his head, pressing his elbows backwards, and arching slightly backwards in the chair, to tighten the chest muscles. Then ask him to take a deep breath, and breathe "on top of this breath" using chest strategies. With the chest muscles tight, this chest breathing is often uncomfortable. Ask the patient to remain in position, but to switch to diaphragmatic breathing by breathing all the way out, then breathing in slowly.

In all cases, it is important to remind the patient that he may feel mildly lightheaded during breathing practice procedures (due to the increased efficiency of the diaphragmatic breath). To help the patient breathe at an appropriately slow pace, you may want to introduce specific timing of breaths. For example, counting "1, 2, 3" during an inhalation and then counting from 1 to 5 during exhalation. Alternatively, subvocalizing the word "Relax" can be used to time breathing. During inhalations the patient should think, "Reeee" and when they exhale, "laaaaaaaaaax."

Breathing skills should be assigned for twice-a-day home practice, with review of procedures during each of the next three sessions (approximately 5 min per session). Because breathing and relaxation strategies are only minor strategies in this treatment, more time generally should not be devoted to these procedures.

Progressive Muscle Relaxation

Progressive muscle relaxation is a useful skill for coping and for promoting tension reduction and a sense of well-being. The relaxation training procedure utilizes repeated tension (10 s) and relaxation (20 s) procedures for a select set of muscle groups (as adapted from Jacobsonian

Progressive Muscle Relaxation.) In addition, a 10-second relaxation cue is taught (in the following session), to aid the in-the-moment application of relaxation procedures.

Progressive Muscle Relaxation Script

You may use the following script to facilitate an 8-muscle group PMR exercise with the patient.

1) Arms Muscle Group

   Build up the tension in your arms by making fists and holding your arms out in front of you with your elbows at a 45-degree angle. Notice the sensations of pulling, discomfort, and tightness in your hands, lower arms, and upper arms. Hold the tension. (Pause 10 s.) *Now release the tension and let your arms and hands relax, with palms facing down. Focus your attention on the sensations of relaxation through your hands, lower arms, and upper arms. As you relax, breathe smoothly and slowly from your abdomen. Each time you exhale, think the word "relax."* (Pause 20 s and then repeat the muscle group for a second practice)

2) Legs Muscle Groups

   Now, build up the tension in your legs by lifting your legs slightly off the floor and, if you feel comfortable, pointing your feet inward. Feel the tension as it moves up your feet into your ankles, shins, calves, and thighs. Feel the pulling sensations from the hip down. Hold the tension. (Pause 10 s.) *Now, release the tension, lowering your legs and relaxing the feet. Feel the warmth and heaviness of relaxation through your feet, lower legs, and upper legs. As you breathe smoothly and slowly, think the word "relax" each time you exhale.* (Pause 20 s and then repeat the muscle group for a second practice.)

3) Stomach Muscle Group

   Now, make your stomach hard by pulling your stomach in toward your spine very tightly. Feel the tightness of your stomach muscles. Focus on that part of your body and hold the tension. (Pause 10 s.)

Now, let your stomach relax outwards. Let it go further and further. Feel the sense of warmth circulating across your stomach. Feel the soft comfort of relaxation. As you breathe smoothly and slowly, think the word "relax" each time you exhale. (Pause 20 s and then repeat the muscle group for a second practice.)

4) Chest Muscle Group

Now, build up the tension around your chest by taking a deep breath and holding it. Your chest is expanded, and the muscles are stretched around it. Feel the tension in your chest and back. Hold your breath. (Pause 10 s.) *Now, slowly, let the air escape and breathe normally, letting the air flow in and out smoothly and easily. Feel the difference as the muscles relax compared with the tension, and think the word "relax" each time you exhale.* (Pause for 20 s and then repeat the muscle group for a second practice.)

5) Shoulders and Upper Back Muscle Group

Pull your shoulder blades back and together. Feel the tension around your shoulders and radiating down into your back. Concentrate on the sensation of tension in this part of your body. (Pause 10 s.) *Now relax your shoulder blades and let them return to a normal position. Focus on the sense of relaxation around your shoulders and across your upper back. Feel the difference in these muscles from the tension. As you breathe smoothly and slowly, think the word "relax" each time you exhale.* (Pause 20 s and then repeat the muscle group for a second practice.)

6) Neck Muscle Group

Build up the tension around your neck by pulling your chin down toward your chest and raising and tightening your shoulders. Feel the tightness around the back of your neck spreading up into the back of your head. Focus on the tension. (Pause 10 s.) *Now, release the tension, letting your head rest comfortably and your shoulders droop. Concentrate on the relaxation. Feel the difference from the tension. As you breathe smoothly and slowly, think the word "relax" each time you exhale.* (Pause 20 s and then repeat the muscle group for a second practice.)

7) Mouth, Jaw, and Throat Muscle Group

Build up the tension around your mouth, jaw, and throat by clenching your teeth and forcing the corners of your mouth back into a forced smile. Feel the tightness, and concentrate on the sensations of tension. (Pause 10 s.) *Then, release the tension, letting your mouth drop open and the muscles around your throat and jaw relax. Concentrate on the difference in the sensations in that part of your body. As you breathe smoothly and slowly, think the word "relax" each time you exhale.* (Pause 20 s and then repeat the muscle group for a second practice.)

8) Eyes and Forehead Muscle Group

Squeeze your eyes tightly shut while pulling your eyebrows down and toward the center. Feel the tension across your lower forehead and around the eyes. Concentrate on the tension. (Pause 10 s.) *Now release, letting the tension around your eyes slide away. Relax the forehead, smoothing out the wrinkles. Feel the difference of relaxation in comparison to tension. As you breathe smoothly and slowly, think the word "relax" each time you exhale.* (Pause 20 s and then repeat the muscle group for a second practice.)

Chapter 21

Anger Management Module

(Corresponds to chapter 14 of the workbook)

Materials Needed

- Thought Record
- Problem-Solving Worksheet

Outline

- Set agenda (as in previous sessions)
- Review Mood Chart (as in previous sessions)
- Review homework (as in previous sessions)
- Introduce anger management
- Conduct behavioral analysis
- Apply cognitive restructuring and problem-solving approaches
- Summarize session (as in previous sessions)
- Assign homework (as in previous sessions)

Introduction to Anger Management

Anger and irritability are relatively common elements of both depressed and (hypo)manic mood states. In depression, irritability and anger may emerge as part of a lower threshold for annoyance and may be part of the patient's sense of not being able to "cope with one more thing." In (hypo)mania, anger and irritability can be part of the internal pressure and sense of urgency that is part of the mood state. With impaired judgment and a heightened sense of importance, the urge to "correct" perceived injustices ("I can't believe they parked there" or "I can't believe my boss has an issue with *that*") may lead to angry outbursts or confrontational behavior. Accordingly, interventions for anger and irritability in bipolar disorder concern not only the management of the aversive mood state of anger, but also attention to reducing the opportunity and the emergence of aggressive or confrontational behaviors that may compromise the patient's longer term goals.

This module of treatment is directed toward helping patients manage their anger and confrontational behaviors more effectively. As with previous sections of this manual, application of new skills is based on an analysis of the chain of thoughts, feelings, and behaviors that preceded episodes of anger. Once maladaptive patterns are identified, the goal is to apply cognitive restructuring and problem-solving approaches (including avoidance of situations where maladaptive confrontations may be likely) to help patients learn alternative reactions to each "choice point" leading up to a potential angry outburst (e.g., each moment when a non-anger inducing behavior or cognition was available for use). In behavioral analysis, the identification of early signs (e.g., a rising voice, muscle tension, and self-defeating thoughts) signaling rising anger is important, given that it is easier to prevent angry outburst before the emergence of extreme feelings of anger.

In preparing a patient for anger management interventions, it is important to clarify for the patient that the goal is to maximize her own feelings of well-being. Anger and aggressive behavior are conceptualized as a problem in its own right; the goal is to reduce anger and reduce the consequences of anger (including aggressive behavior and further exacerbations in mood state). The goal is not to debate the relevance of cues for anger (e.g., "can you believe my spouse did that" or "who drives like that"), but to frame the issue as follows: "Regardless of the immediate reasons for your feelings of anger, our goal in therapy is to help you better manage your anger as part of your management of bipolar disorder."

Behavioral Analysis

The first step in anger management is conducting a step-by-step analysis of the event that made the patient angry, irritable, or frustrated. It is imperative to identify as many thoughts, behaviors, and feelings that preceded the angry outburst as possible. It is important to write down what the patient reports, tracking the cascade of thoughts, feelings, and behaviors leading up to an episode of anger or aggressive behavior.

The following case vignette illustrates aspects of the behavioral analysis used to identify initial targets for intervention for cognitive restructuring and problem solving:

Case Vignette

P: Well, I lost it again. I began yelling at my girlfriend on the phone, and then she hung up on me and I got so mad that I threw a cup across the room. I hate it when I get that way. It feels like I've got no control and that I'm losing my mind.

T: Let's see if we can figure out some ways to help you. Describe the situation to me in as much detail as possible. Begin with what was happening before the call came.

P: Well, nothing really. I was just watching the game.

T: What were you thinking?

P: That the team sucked! They were blowing their lead! I was so mad at them. I was leaping out of the chair yelling at the TV.

T: So, before the call from your girlfriend came, you were already angry, jumping up and down, and thinking negative thoughts about the game.

P: Yeah, I practically lunged at the phone and yelled, "Hello!" when she called.

T: So, I wonder if you could have waited a bit before you picked up the phone. You could have waited until the phone rang a bit, or even let the answering machine pick up the call. What happened when you picked up the phone?

P: Oh man! She started again with her nagging about how I don't spend enough time with her and all I do is watch sports. I mean, I spend so much time with her already. Can't I just watch a game every now and then? It's not like I haven't asked her to watch it with me, but she doesn't like sports that much.

T: I don't want to get into who was right, since your girlfriend is not here. I want to help you manage your anger so you don't start yelling, which you said is a problem.

P: Yeah, it is. I don't like doing that to her or anyone.

T: So, what were you doing when she starting telling you that you were not spending enough time with her?

P: I got quiet. I always do. And then I started to shake my head and next thing you know I'm pacing back and forth in my apartment. And then I lost it.

T: OK. What were you thinking when the conversation started?

P: "Here we go again." You know, my previous girlfriend used to nag all the time. I mean all the time. She's not as bad as the other one was. She just gets upset with this issue.

T: So, when your current girlfriend told you that she was upset, you right away thought about your previous girlfriend and all the nagging she used to do. What were you feeling during the conversation?

P: I just got angry.

T: Do you think there was anything else you might have felt just before you got angry?

P: Well, I was frustrated because I wanted to watch the game. I also felt guilty because I told her that I wasn't going to watch the game that day, but was going to clean my car. I think I felt like a little kid who was caught. But, it's not like we're married. She needs to relax!

T: So, we've identified that you were feeling frustrated and guilty before you became angry. You also thought that this situation was similar to your past girlfriend. Finally, you became quiet, shook your head, and then started pacing before you yelled. Do I have it right?

P: Sounds right to me.

T: So, it seems that you have some warning signs that you need to be more aware of. For example, when you begin to get quiet, that is a sign that you are getting frustrated or irritable. Or, when you begin to get memories of your past girlfriend's nagging, that might a good time to check in with yourself and ask, "is this really that similar?" or "do I really want to pile together my memories of being frustrated in the past with what I am feeling now?"

P: It just seems to happen so fast, when I get angry.

T: Well, this is one reason why we want to find your specific warning bells for anger, so that you can intervene right away. In particular, I would like you to use the Thought Record this week to identify thoughts that tend to increase anger. If we can help you react differently to these thoughts, then we should give you a bit more power over your angry reactions.

Cognitive Restructuring

For cognitive restructuring of episodes of anger, therapists should attend to some of the classic thoughts associated with anger. In particular, in the preceding dialogue, the patient was able to identify two immediate targets for cognitive intervention:

1. "I also felt guilty because . . . I felt like a little kid who was caught"

2. "Here we go again" (this is just like the pattern with my past girlfriend).

The latter thought, "here we go again" is a classic target for anger management, where the patient brings forward past frustrations into the current situations, thereby intensifying the emotion and the perceived need to respond. Other cognitions consistent with this theme include:

- This is just like last time.

- He is always doing this to me.

- Here we go again; this is endless.

Other classic cognitions associated with anger concern personalizing a perceived offense:

- He is doing this on purpose, to mess with me.

- He thinks my feelings are unimportant

- He has no respect for me.

The natural thought in response for these intensifying cognitions is

- I have to put a stop to this.

- People can't just continue to mess with me

- No one should have to take this.

Any and all of these cognitions are good targets for intervention in helping patients better try to coach themselves away from anger and aggression intensifying cognitions.

Problem Solving

In addition to cognitive interventions for anger, therapists should also attend to what problem-solving action needs to be adopted by the patient. That is, in studies of anger management, both social skill training and training in problem solving offers reliable benefit. Accordingly, use of the Problem-Solving Worksheet (see Chapter 17) and assertiveness training (see Chapter 18) should be applied in conjunction with cognitive interventions. Also, therapists need to plan for the management of conflict when there is a lowered threshold to irritability and aggressive outbursts during hypomanic or manic episodes. During this time, the most valuable intervention may be to help the patient minimize opportunities for escalation of anger into aggressive behavior. That is, both therapists and patients need to recognize periods when self-defeating confrontational behavior by the patient is at a high probability, and to use selective avoidance (until better skills can be developed) to protect the patient's self interests until the irritable mood resolves. In short, therapists may want to ask patients to "invest in their future" by being a good manager of themselves during periods of irritability with the goal of reducing opportunities for damaging arguments in high-risk work and family events or meetings. An example of this intervention follows.

Case Vignette

T: And so we see by your Mood Chart that you are fighting a lot of irritability right now, and you also have a number of symptoms of hypomania.

P: Yeah. Before coming here I almost screamed at my husband. I am already feeling like I am coping with as much stuff as I can, and he just had to talk about the weekend plans and all he wants to get done. And I could not tell whether he was really being annoying on purpose or whether it was the irritability, so I just got the heck out before I blew. But I also felt like not coming here, thinking that I might be yelling at you during the session

T: I am glad you came, let's see how we do with your irritability today. But also, I think the option you selected with your husband is valuable for you. You have talked before how much you regret the arguments you and your husband have when you are irritable. Today, you prevented one such argument by just getting out of the house.

P: Yeah, but I can't believe he just *has* to talk about all the plans, right when I am just trying to hold it together.

T: There are at least three issues here. The first is to work on a plan for how you and your husband discuss weekends and other "to do" times. The second is for us to continue to work on how to manage irritability so that it is less distressing to you. And the third is to ensure that, while we are building your skills with irritability, you don't have arguments or confrontations that you don't want to have, especially when you look back on this period after your mood resolves.

P: Yeah, I hate all that regret.

T: OK, let's start with how to avoid arguments and confrontations. Are there ways we can help you minimize the opportunity for "blowups" at home while you work with me and your pharmacotherapist on more broadly managing this hypomanic period?

P: Well, I can't avoid everything.

T: Right, but let's talk through your schedule for this week. Are there any situations or times when you think it might be especially hard to keep your irritability in check?

P: Saturday morning is always rough. There is so much bustle with the weekend agenda and the kids. I can really see that going badly.

T: Just for this week, are there alternatives you can identify for how to handle the initial 2–3 hr period of Saturday morning?

P: It would be so much better to just go off and have coffee by myself and then start the day later.

T: How would that play with your husband?

P: He would probably do anything not to have another Saturday argument—it hurts the whole weekend. Everyone walks around on eggshells then. I hate it.

T: Ok. One goal might be to have you talk with your husband so that he understands fully what is going on. You may want to say something like, "I really am having a tough week with my frustration and irritability, and you know how much I hate it when I blow up at you or the kids. I am thinking that it might be a better way for us to start the weekend if I go off by myself Saturday morning, and then try to engage better with you and the kids later in the day. How would that plan be for you?"

P: That is interesting. I usually don't explain it to him like that. He might like that. He says he is just looking for some sense of control when I get this way.

T: OK, let's do two things. Let's first do a role play of you actually requesting this change here in the session. Then, let's also talk about other things you can do to manage your irritability during this time period.

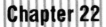

Chapter 22 | *Managing Extreme Emotions Module*

Therapist Note

■ *This module is only for patients who suffer repeated crisis situations and need short-term coping strategies.* ■

There are no materials needed

Outline

- ■ Set agenda (as in previous sessions)

- ■ Review Mood Chart (as in previous sessions)

- ■ Review homework (as in previous sessions)

- ■ Introduce the management of extreme emotions

- ■ Discuss the role of acceptance

- ■ Teach distraction techniques

- ■ Teach awareness skills

- ■ Summarize session (as in previous sessions)

- ■ Assign homework (as in previous sessions)

Introduction to the Management of Extreme Emotions

Mood swings are inherent in bipolar disorder, and patients often have a difficult time coping with the mood swings, leading to anxiety or a worsening of a mood state. Comorbid Axis II disorders may also contribute to extreme mood states and a lowered ability to use other coping strategies. Although the primary focus of treatment is to help patients develop more optimal methods of coping with problems, occasionally moments arise when patients feel overwhelmed by emotion. Under these conditions, a patient may need alternative, short-term strategies for coping.

This module is designed to provide patients with strategies for short-term coping with extreme feelings and moods. These strategies are drawn from Linehan's (1993) *Congnitive-Behavioral Treatment of Borderline Personality Disorder*. This module of treatment should not be used with every patient, but is instead saved for those individuals who suffer repeated crisis situations. That is, active problem solving, contacting treatment providers when in crisis, or challenging dysfunctional cognitions should remain the primary way that a patient handles his difficulties. However, there will be times when outside interventions and supports will be unavailable or when the patient's methods for coping are ineffective for the demands of a situation. It is at these moments that managing more difficult emotions is appropriate. It is up to you and the patient to determine when an emotion is simply "too hot" to examine, and when other skills are warranted so that the situation can be reexamined later when things "cool down."

Role of Acceptance

At times, the best that a patient can do in a difficult situation is to accept reality and cope with the subsequent emotions. For example, many bipolar patients in a manic phase have lost jobs, have made poor financial decisions, or have inadvertently damaged relationships with loved ones. The emotional fallout from those experiences can be great. Similarly, many patients in the depressed phase feel so overwhelmed with negative emotions and suicidal ideation that coping from day-to-day is an enormous struggle. It is in these situations and others that distress tolerance skills are useful for the bipolar patient, along with active problem solving, treatment adherence, and bridging interpersonal or communication problems. At times, the patient must accept that a relationship may be beyond repair, a recent manic episode has caused enormous consequences both professionally and financially, or that he has a chronic illness that will not simply go away. The subsequent emotions that go with accepting these situations often are difficult to manage for the bipolar patient.

Distraction Techniques

One effective tool for managing difficult emotions is distraction. Explain to the patient that by distraction, you do not mean ignoring a problem or wishing it away. Distracting entails an active effort on the patient's part to deflect the intensity of emotional experiences *in order to find and implement solutions later.* For example, engaging in some sort of activity when emotions become overwhelming is a good distraction strategy. Taking a walk, cleaning a room, calling a friend, exercising, watching children play, etc. can help the patient defuse his negative mood state so that he can have a better perspective on a situation.

Patients who are more depressed and who are having acute difficulties engaging in any activity can use techniques to distract themselves from their thoughts. For example, asking a patient to count items, describe a painting, imagine his favorite vacation spot, etc. can help him distract himself from his intense feelings until he can implement a more thorough plan later.

A key point with distraction skills is that the patient should not try to make an intense thought "go away." Distraction techniques introduce new, competing thoughts to the ones that are overwhelming or intense. In this manner, the patient begins to calm himself by staying focused on the new thoughts and actions.

Case Vignette 1

This case vignette illustrates when to ask the patient to use distraction techniques:

P: You know, I just kept on trying to solve that problem. I went at it and at it from different angles. I thought I was going to scream. After about my 10th try, I gave up and then all those negative thoughts we had talked about came out. It was a mess!

T: I wonder if you could have kept your mind clearer and your emotions more in check if you would have taken a walk around the office after the 2nd or 3rd try with the problem.

P: Yeah, but that doesn't solve the problem I had.

T: You're right, it won't solve the problem you were working on, but it allows you to accept that you're having a tough time and it gives your mind a break. By distracting yourself for a few moments, you will be able to return to your problem and have a clearer perspective.

P: Yeah, I was so wound up in my mood that I thought the only way out was to keep on trying harder.

T: Exactly! Another way around your mood may have been to take a short break, give yourself a few minutes to think of something else, and then return to the problem.

Case Vignette 2

The depressed patient may pose a different set of problems when trying to implement distraction techniques. As in this case vignette, simple distraction from thoughts can be helpful.

P: I was stuck in "depression land" this past week. I found out that my company fired me after I said all those things to my coworkers when I was manic. I just didn't know what to do after I got that call. It was overwhelming. It seemed like all my coping skills just flew out the window.

T: I think anyone would be sad and upset over that news. What did you do after you found out the news?

P: I didn't do anything. I just lay on my couch and obsessed about how crappy my life is. And then I started to tell myself that I hated my life. I just kept on thinking that I wish I were dead. I tried to get my friend, Susan, on the phone like we talked about, but she wasn't home yet from work. I just kept on thinking about how horrible things are and I cried for 2 hours. I couldn't stop crying.

T: Do you think there could have been something else you could have thought about besides the loss of your job until Susan came home?

P: Like what?

T: Like doing simple distractions like counting or reciting something out loud. Anything to distract your mind from your overwhelming feeling. Maybe even watch TV.

P: I just found out that my job is not taking me back and you want me to watch soap operas?

T: These are things to do when all else fails. You can't get your job back, Susan won't be home for 2 hours, and you're feeling so overwhelmed that you cannot stop crying. You need to get your mind off of your thoughts. So, yeah, watching some bad soap opera might be enough of a distraction to get you through that difficult period. Counting, reading a mindless magazine, or anything to help distract you enough to help you tolerate the intense feelings.

Awareness Skills

The patient can also manage difficult emotions by simply being more aware of the moment. By being more aware, the patient becomes more attuned to the world around him and less attuned to his emotional pain. This technique is similar to distraction techniques, but it requires that the patient become more centered and present focused.

One way for the patient to become more present focused is to have him check in with his environment through his senses. Using this method often gets the patient out of his feeling state as he is focusing attention on his immediate environment and not on his difficult mood state. By focusing on the immediate environment and the information that is being picked up by his senses, the patient will be focused less on his disturbing experiences and more on the world around him. This technique is similar to the skills trauma victims use when they are attempting to stop dissociative episodes. Though the emotional experiences might be less intense than trauma victims, the skills are applicable to the patient with bipolar disorder.

The case vignette that follows exemplifies how to teach skills of awareness. To be able to apply this skill at home, the patient may need to practice these techniques when in a normal mood state. If there is evidence that the patient has repeated difficulties with managing extreme emotions, assign regular rehearsal of awareness strategies.

Case Vignette

P: I got some real bad news today. I received my credit card bill in the mail and I owe $25,000. I don't know what I'm going to do. I'm so overwhelmed with my feelings right now that I barely made it here today and I want to start crying and screaming. *(Patient begins crying.)* How could this happen? I can't repay this! What should I do?

T: Well, we could try to problem solve this dilemma, but right now it seems that your feelings are getting the better of you. This gives us a good opportunity to practice some ways you can calm down. You're right, $25,000 is a lot of money, and I wish we could make it go away, but we can't. So, let me teach you some ways to cope until we can figure out a plan.

P: OK.

T: I'm going to teach you some skills for becoming more aware of your environment so that you can focus more on what is going around you, and less on your problems or emotions. OK? First, I want you to describe my office to me. Tell me every detail that you can.

P: *(Patient describes color of walls, number of bookshelves, paintings in the room, items on the desk, etc.)*

T: Now, I want you to describe the sounds in this office. Take a few moments and listen for all the sounds that you hear, and describe them to me.

P: *(Patient describes the hum of the fan, the people talking in the hallway, the noise from the computer, etc.)*

T: Now, I want you to describe the sensations on your body.

P: *(Patient describes sitting in the chair, crossing his legs, etc.)*

T: Now, how do you feel?

P: Better.

T: Good! What you just did was calm yourself down. The problem is still there, but your feelings are more under your control. Now let's figure out some ways we can manage your financial problems.

Treatment Phase 4

Chapter 23 | *Well-Being Therapy and Relapse Prevention*

(Corresponds to chapter 15 of the workbook)

Materials Needed

- Review Worksheets

Outline

- Set agenda (as in previous sessions)

- Review Mood Chart (as in previous sessions)

- Review homework (as in previous sessions)

- Introduce a well-being therapy approach

- Help the patient define her "purpose" in life

- Review the patient's well-being diary

- Return to therapist training for the patient

- Discuss relapse prevention

- Conclude therapy

Framework for Well-Being Therapy

In the final phase of treatment, the methods of treatment remain largely the same but the target for intervention shifts from symptom reduction to the attainment of well-being. The conceptual framework for this approach is based on Ryff and Singer's (1996) model of psychological well-being and is encouraged by recent investigation of the application of this model to relapse prevention (Fava, 1999; Fava & Ruini, 2003; Fava et al., 1998). Enduring recovery, according to Ryff and Singer, is hastened by a direct focus on engendering positive patterns. That is, the absence of well-being is viewed as a risk factor for future difficulties. Nonetheless, they argue that the removal of problematic patterns is not the same as engendering positive ones. As such, Ryff and Singer break with mental health's traditional focus on the amelioration of dysfunction and instead target the attainment and maintenance of periods of well-being.

The therapeutic tools utilized in well-being therapy are the traditional tools of cognitive-behavioral therapy (CBT) and will be immediately recognizable by readers of this manual: (1) cognitive restructuring, (2) activity management (targeting mastery, pleasure, and skill development), (3) assertiveness training, and (4) problem solving.

Format for Well-Being Therapy

Fava (1999) describes a multi-phase format for well-being therapy, with sessions (weekly or biweekly) organized into three complementary stages. In the first stage, the patient is asked to keep a structured diary of periods of well-being (a sort of "hedonic book keeping"). In the second stage, monitoring is shifted to include automatic thoughts surrounding periods of well-being. Unlike the procedures used thus far in this manual, the triggers for the patient's self-monitoring are periods of well-being rather than periods of distress. The task is to attend to periods of well-being, enjoy them, and attend to cognitions or other events which may interfere with ongoing enjoyment. In the third stage, the therapist intervenes with cognitive restructuring, activity assignments, and skills training to help the patient better maximize periods of well-being. In this stage, the therapist is guided by a conceptual framework defining domains where well-being can be enhanced (see Fava, 1999, pp. 173–174). These areas include:

(1)   mastery over one's environment, including selection of situations and activities that promote well-being;

(2)   personal growth, including a sense of realizing one's own potential and the development of additional skills and valued aspects of the self over time;

(3)   purpose in life, including, if needed, a clear restatement aims, values, and objectives for living;

(4)   autonomy, including the ability to resist social pressures and use personal standards for evaluation;

(5)   self-acceptance, including identification and acceptance of one's good and bad qualities and past deeds;

(6)   positive relationships with others, including the capability to have strong empathy, affection, and intimacy, as well as an understanding of the give and take of human relationships.

In relation to these key concepts, it is clear that the problem-list phase of treatment (Phase 3) provides a wealth of skills for well-being interventions. For example, training in goal setting, problem solving, assertiveness, and scheduling of pleasant events are strategies that are richly compatible with most of the key concepts just listed. This phase of treatment, however, focuses more directly on accentuating what is "working" by trying to extend periods of well-being.

For the application of a well-being approach to bipolar patients, some care needs to be taken in defining the outcome of treatment. The goal is to increase stable, positive affective states. These states need to be differentiated from the overpositive thoughts, euphoria, and overactivity characteristic of hypomanic states. Instead the target is the maximization of stable periods of well-being.

Because the application of well-being therapy in this protocol concerns the targets rather than the strategies of treatment, it can be applied at any point the patient is in remission. Accordingly, elements of a well-being approach to treatment can be initiated anytime during the last eight sessions of this protocol, as long as the patient is in remission. However, even if the patient is not in remission, a well-being focus should be incorporated into ongoing treatment efforts for at least the last four sessions (Sessions 27–30). These sessions occur biweekly. This schedule of biweekly appointments (initiated at Session 21) allows the patient to have more time practicing skills independent of the therapist, and allows treatment to fade gradually. During this time, one explicit goal is for the patient to fully adopt the role of the therapist, reviewing her diary, examining her strategies, and assigning relevant skill rehearsal to improve well-being. Over these sessions, the therapist increasingly plays the role of therapy supervisor, encouraging the patient in her application of therapy skills.

Introducing a Well-Being Approach

When the patient is reliably euthymic, or when Session 27 has been reached, introduce a well-being focus. This introduction should make it clear that a focus on pleasure is the natural endpoint to all therapies, and that the shift in treatment simply reflects a more-direct focus on increasing the positive rather than removing the negative. For example, you may say something like the following:

> *During the last few months, you have learned a great deal about using cognitive-behavioral therapy to decrease patterns that do not serve you well. In our work together, we have devoted time to* (list major targets in treatment thus far). *However, to complement this work on decreasing problematic patterns, we should also spend some time on increasing positive patterns and feelings of well-being. As part of each of the remaining sessions of our planned treatment, I want to make sure that we spend time focusing on increasing pleasure, and locking in the habit of using cognitive-behavioral skills to maximize enjoyment in your life.*

Defining "Purpose"

For the focus on well-being it is helpful to have a clear, overarching definition of meaning in life from the patient. This definition can then be used as an ultimate standard for organizing targets for greater well-being. The goal is simply to help the patient examine her own definitions of meaning and purpose, and then use this definition to judge the appropriateness of maladaptive behaviors.

You will need to use your judgment about when to introduce an intervention around "purpose." That is, if the patient is extremely pessimistic, you may want to restrict this discussion to in session, where pessimistic attitudes can be identified and restructured. However, for most patients, questions about meaning can be assigned as a home practice assignment. For example, you may say:

> As we prepare to have you focus more on increasing pleasure, I want to make sure that I get a clear definition from you of what you think is valuable in life. In short, I am going to ask you to provide me with a definition of the "purpose" of life for you. What is it all about? What are you supposed to do while you are alive? And what is the role of fun, of work, of relationships? I want to make sure that you are guiding yourself effectively around those things that you think are really important. Next session, I would like you to define for me the purpose for or meaning in life. I would like you to approach this task like you are giving me advice on how to live my life, what is important. Does this sound OK?

In most cases, the patient returns to the next session with a description of the importance of:

- productivity (to make a difference)

- connection or bond with others (to love)

- pleasure (to have some fun)

Patients may differ wildly on how these domains of meaning are defined and the degree to which religious issues predominate. It is your goal to facilitate the patient's unique statement of meaning, and then to use this overarching goal structure to help the patient plan well-being interventions. For example, you may say:

> So, when we take a look at your self-monitoring, we should ask whether some of the old habits (cognitions) you have serve you well or not for these goals for life. For example, you have long been extremely self-critical. Can you tell me whether the self-criticism helps with these goals, or whether it is just a left-over habit that does not tend to serve you well?

The primary purpose of the well-being diary is to help the patient recognize and attend to periods of well-being. Instruct the patient to buy a small bound notebook or journal that she finds attractive. The patient will use this diary to record daily episodes of well-being.

> *Every day, I want you to record the moment of the day when you felt the most well-being; even on sad days, I want you to think back over the day, and pick out the best moment and record it.*

In addition to recording the situation or event associated with well-being, the patient should record the cognitions and feelings accompanying the particular episode. In reviewing this assignment, you should be oriented to "sharing the joy" of these moments by having the patient explain what was pleasurable about the events. Your nonverbal communication is important during this review, and you should show eager involvement in the patient's description of pleasant events. Review of the diary should be followed by an open discussion of what can be done in the next week to continue periods of well-being.

After one to two sessions have been devoted to reviews of this kind, greater attention can be devoted to identification of cognitions or events that block the planning or sustained enjoyment of periods of well-being. This self-monitoring and subsequent problem solving is nearly identical to the problem-list phase of treatment, except that the target for monitoring and problem solving is periods of well-being.

Further Therapist Training for the Patient

As the final several sessions approach, you should return attention to the patient's "therapist training." Therapist training was utilized in Session 1 to help the patient adopt a therapeutic attitude toward herself and her problems. In the final sessions of treatment, the patient is asked to take more and more responsibility for independently directing the problem solving and skill rehearsal elements of CBT. For example you might say:

Therapy will continue on its current topics: a review of what went well over the last week, blocks to well-being, and a problem-solving focus on how you can better enjoy the week and meet your goals. Next week, I would like you to hold a session at our regular time, but do it at home, by yourself. You know by now my approach, how we structure the session, and the feel of focusing on your current patterns with the goal of increasing well-being. I want you to run next session yourself, and then I want you to come see me in 2 weeks. We will then spend sometime reviewing how you did acting as the only therapist on the case.
I will play the role of therapy supervisor and ask you how your patient is doing, and how you are directing her therapy. How does this sound?

Relapse-Prevention Readiness—The Final Session

The final session of treatment is devoted to review and extension of therapy principles. To aid the patient in further developing a model of what has been successful in her treatment, you should recap each of the patient's accomplishments in therapy, with a specific review of strategies that appeared to help the patient. This review should next transition to a more formal discussion of relapse-prevention skills using the Review Worksheets in the workbook (copies for your use are provided in the appendix). For example, you may say:

Sometime in the future, I don't know when, I know that you will have a downturn of mood for several days. Nothing will seem to be going well, and you will feel sad and tired. I am saying this is going to happen, because I think it happens to everyone. When you have your downturn, what things do you want to remind yourself about, or what skills do you want to apply to help this downturn last only a short time?

Discuss the patient's skills and expectations. Have her record her relapse-prevention strategies on the worksheet. This is a list of the skills and interventions that the patient has experienced as being helpful, as well as skills relevant to the vulnerability areas the patient identified. You may end the discussion with the following dialogue:

My own model of treatment is that therapy never ends; it is just that patients learn to conduct the therapy for themselves. You have really done well adopting a therapeutic perspective and working as your own therapist. I want you to continue this approach, and to continue your focus on helping yourself experience well-being. Remember that as a tool to help you remember some of the topic areas for therapy, you have your workbook. It will be helpful if you review this workbook occasionally to make sure your therapy stays on track. In addition, you should also review the Relapse Prevention Worksheet in your workbook to remind yourself to use cognitive-behavioral strategies when you need them.

Concluding Therapy

Given the chronic and cyclic nature of bipolar disorder, individuals with this disorder may not be free of the need for continued therapy. Therefore, the therapist should communicate a sense of completion of a stage of therapy relevant to a stage of the disorder. In all cases, patients should be encouraged to return to therapy as the course of their bipolar disorder demands. Use of separate epochs of treatment may help patients consolidate treatment gains and expand self-therapy skills. If individuals should elect to return for additional treatment, use of the problem-list phase as part of assessment can be useful for resetting goals for the next epoch of care.

Appendix of Forms

Core Belief Worksheet

Situation:	Thought:	Feeling:
Theme behind this thought:		

Situation:	Thought:	Feeling:
Theme behind this thought:		

Potential Core Belief:

Core Strategies

Age:	Situation:
Belief Formed From This Event	
Strategy for Dealing With The Event	

Age:	Situation:
Belief Formed From This Event	
Strategy for Dealing With The Event	

Age:	Situation:
Belief Formed From This Event	
Strategy for Dealing With The Event	

Source: Form based on strategies in Beck, J. S. (1995). Cognitive theraphy: Basics and beyond. New York: Guilford.

Problem-Solving Worksheet

What is the problem:

_____

Why does this problem bother me (what are the specific features that bother me)?

_____

_____

_____

Is this a realistic problem (e.g., what do I really think is going to happen, and what part of this problem do I think is just worry)?

_____

How can I rewrite the problem clearly, so that it helps me think about a solution? Write in a clear restatement of the problem:

_____

_____

Now that I have the problem clearly in mind, what are potential solutions to this problem? To generate solutions, I want to think about as many possible solutions as possible (without thinking why they are good or bad, and without choosing an option at this point). What advice might a good friend give? If a friend had this problem, what advice would I give?

Potential options:

_____

_____

_____

_____

_____

_____

Now rate each potential option. For each option rate the good and bad aspects of the proposed solution. Do not select an option until each is rated.

Good things about each solution   Bad things about each solution

1.

2.

3.

4.

5.

6.

Given this evaluation, which solution seems best?

_____

Do you want to apply this solution, or is more time or more information needed to solve this problem?

_____

Problem-Solving Worksheet

What is the problem:

Arguments with my spouse about money

Why does this problem bother me (what are the specific features that bother me)?

I want a better sense of control over our finances.

I feel like I'm the only one who really cares what happens with our money.

Is this a realistic problem (e.g., what do I really think is going to happen, and what part of this problem do I think is just worry)?

Yes, we really argue quite often about money

How can I rewrite the problem clearly, so that it helps me think about a solution? Write in a clear restatement of the problem:

My spouse and I don't plan how to spend money, and then we're surprised by what each of us has spent. This always leads to an argument.

Now that I have the problem clearly in mind, what are potential solutions to this problem? To generate solutions, I want to think about as many possible solutions as possible (without thinking why they are good or bad, and without choosing an option at this point). What advice might a good friend give? If a friend had this problem, what advice would I give?

Potential options:

1. Just keep doing what we're doing.

2. Set up a weekly meeting where my spouse and I can discuss our finances and the household budget.

3. Open separate bank accounts.

4. Use a notebook to track expenses and review with one another on a weekly basis.

5. Assign a small amount of money as "free use" money and create a stricter budget for managing the rest.

continued

Now rate each potential option. For each option rate the good and bad aspects of the proposed solution. Do not select an option until each is rated.

Good things about each solution   Bad things about each solution

1. No effort required   Nothing is resolved and things may get worse

2. Gives us a chance to talk openly about money   We may end up fighting during meetings

3. Gives each of us a sense of freedom   I would feel like we aren't partners

4. Makes each of us accountable and makes sure we talk to each other about money   May be hard to remember to use the notebook

5. Like option #3, this gives us more freedom   We really should be buying things together, as a couple

Given this evaluation, which solution seems best?

Options 2 and 4 seem like the best solutions. Tracking our finances and meeting weekly seems to be a good way to start changing the situation.

Do you want to apply this solution, or is more time or more information needed to solve this problem?

Yes, I think we can start having meetings and using a notebook to track our finances. I really want to change things and avoid arguments over money.

228

1-Month Review Sheet

Date of Review _____

1. What skills have you been practicing well, and how are you coaching yourself?

_____

_____

_____

2. Where do you still have troubles, and what concerns do you have about these troubles?

_____

_____

_____

3. What skills do you need to practice?

_____

_____

_____

4. List your treatment goals for the next several months.

_____

_____

_____

5. What positive events are you going to plan so that you have pleasant memories to look back on? Remember that even small events can go a long way toward increasing happiness.

_____

_____

_____

3-Month Review Sheet

Date of Review _____

1. What skills have you been practicing well, and how are you coaching yourself?

_____

_____

_____

2. Where do you still have troubles, and what concerns do you have about these troubles?

_____

_____

_____

3. What skills do you need to practice?

_____

_____

_____

4. List your treatment goals for the next several months.

_____

_____

_____

5. What positive events are you going to plan so that you have pleasant memories to look back on? Remember that even small events can go a long way toward increasing happiness.

_____

_____

_____

6-Month Review Sheet

Date of Review _____

1. What skills have you been practicing well, and how are you coaching yourself?

_____

_____

_____

2. Where do you still have troubles, and what concerns do you have about these troubles?

_____

_____

_____

3. What skills do you need to practice?

_____

_____

_____

4. List your treatment goals for the next several months.

_____

_____

_____

5. What positive events are you going to plan so that you have pleasant memories to look back on? Remember that even small events can go a long way toward increasing happiness.

_____

_____

_____

Long-Term Goal Sheet

Long-term goal:

_____

_____

_____

Short-term goal:

Skill needed to achieve this goal:

Short-term goal:

Skill needed to achieve this goal:

Short-term goal:

Skill needed to achieve this goal:

Short-term goal:

Skill needed to achieve this goal:

Short-term goal:

Skill needed to achieve this goal:

NOW Your current situation: _____

_____

_____

References

Akiskal, H. S. (2007). The emergence of the bipolar spectrum: Validation along clinical-epidemiologic and familial-genetic lines. *Psychopharmacology Bulletin, 40,* 99–115.

American Psychiatric Association (2000). *Diagnostic and statistical manual of mental disorders* (4th ed., Text Revision). Washington, DC: Author.

Beck, A. T., Steer, R. A., & Brown, G. K. (1996). *Beck depression inventory manual* (2nd ed.). San Antonio: The Psychological Corporation.

Beck, A. T., Weissman, A., Lester, D., & Trexler, L. (1974). The measurement of pessimism: The hopelessness scale. *Journal of Consulting and Clinical Psychology, 42,* 861–865.

Brown, G. K., Beck, A. T., Steer, R. A., & Grisham, J. R. (2000). Risk factors for suicide in psychiatric outpatients: A 20-year prospective study. *Journal of Consulting and Clinical Psychology, 68,* 371–377.

Burns, D. (1999). *Feeling good: The new mood therapy.* New York: Harper Collins.

Cochran, S. D. (1984). Preventing medical noncompliance in the outpatient treatment of bipolar affective disorders. *Journal of Consulting and Clinical Psychology, 52,* 873–878.

Craske, M. G., & Barlow, D. H. (2006). *Mastery of your anxiety and panic, therapist guide* (4th ed.). New York: Oxford University Press.

Dent, J. & Teasdale, J. D. (1988). Negative cognitions and the persistence of depression. *Journal of Abnormal Psychology, 97,* 29–34.

Ellicott, A., Hammen, C., Gitlin, M., Brown, G., & Jamison, K. (1990). Life events and the course of bipolar disorder. *American Journal of Psychiatry, 147,* 1194–1198.

Fava, G. A. (1999). Well-being therapy: Conceptual and technical issues. *Psychotherapy and Psychosomatics, 68,* 171–179.

Fava, G. A., Rafanelli, C., Cazzaro, M., Conti, S., & Grandi, S. (1998). Well-being therapy: A novel psychotherapeutic approach for residual symptoms of affective disorders. *Psychological Medicine, 28,* 475–480.

Fava, G. A., & Ruini, C. 2003 Development and characteristics of a well-being enhancing psychotherapeutic strategy: Well-being therapy. *Journal of Behavior Therapy and Experimental Psychiatry, 34,* 45–63.

First, M. B., Spitzer, R. L., Gibbon, M., & Williams, J. B. W. (2002). *Structured clinical interview for DSM-IV-TR Axis I disorders, research Version, patient edition with psychotic screen (SCID-I/p W/ PSY SCREEN).* New York: Biometrics Research, New York State Psychiatric Institute.

Foa, E. B., & Kozak, M. J. (2004). *Mastery of obsessive-compulsive disorder: A cognitive-behavioral approach, therapist guide.* New York: Oxford University Press.

Frank, E., Hlastala, S., Ritenour, A., Houck, P., Tu, X. M., Monk, T. H. et al. (1997). Inducing lifestyle regularity in recovering bipolar disorder patients: Results from the maintenance therapies in bipolar disorder protocol. *Biological Psychiatry, 41,* 1165–1173.

Frank, E., Swartz, H. A., & Kupfer, D. J. (2000). Interpersonal and social rhythm therapy: Managing the chaos of bipolar disorder. *Biological Psychiatry, 48,* 593–604.

Goldberg, J., Garno, J., Leon, A., Kocsis, J., & Portera, L. (1999). A history of substance abuse complicates remission from acute mania in bipolar disorder. *Journal of Clinical Psychiatry, 60,* 733–740.

Goldberg, J. F., Harrow, M., & Whiteside, R. E. (2001). Risk for bipolar illness in patients initially hospitalized for unipolar depression. *American Journal of Psychiatry, 158,* 1265–1270.

Hayes, S. C., Strosahl, K. D., & Wilson, K. G. (1999). *Acceptance and Commitment Therapy.* New York: Guilford Press.

Henin, A., Otto, M. W., & Reilly-Harrington, N. A. (2001). Introducing flexibility in manualized treatment: Application of recommended strategies to the cognitive-behavioral treatment of bipolar disorder. *Cognitive and Behavioral Practice, 8,* 317–328.

Henry, C., Van den Bulke, D., Bellivier, F., Etan, B., Rouillon, F., & Leboyer, M. (2003). Anxiety disorders in 318 bipolar patients: Prevalence and impact on illness severity and response to mood stabilizer. *Journal of Clinical Psychiatry, 64,* 331–335.

Jamison, K. R. (1997). *An unquiet mind: A memoir of moods and madness.* New York: Vintage.

Johnson, S. L., & Miller, I. (1997). Negative life events and time to recovery from episodes of bipolar disorder. *Journal of Abnormal Psychology, 106,* 449–457.

Judd, L. L., Akiskal, H. S., Schettler, P. J., Coryell, W., Endicott, J., Maser, J. D. et al. (2003). Prospective investigation of the natural history of the long-term weekly symptomatic status of bipolar II disorder. *Archives of General Psychiatry, 60,* 261–269.

Judd, L. L., Akiskal, H. S., Schettler, P. J., Endicott, J., Maser, J. D., Solomon, D. A. et al. (2003). The long-term natural history of the weekly symptomatic status of bipolar I disorder. *Archives of General Psychiatry, 59,* 530–537.

Kahn, D. A., Keck, P. E., Perlis, R. H., Otto, M. W., & Ross, R. (2004 December). Treatment of bipolar disorder: A guide for patients and families. *A Postgraduate Medicine Special Report,* 1–108.

Keck, P. E., McElroy, S. L., Strakowski, S. M., Stanton, S. P., Kizer, D. L., Balistreri, T. M. et al. (1996). Factors associated with pharmacologic noncompliance in patients with mania. *Journal of Clinical Psychiatry, 57,* 292–297.

Keck, P. E. Jr, McElroy, S. L., Strakowski, S. M., West, S. A., Sax, K. W., Hawkins, J. M. et al. (1998). Twelve-month outcome of patients with bipolar disorder following hospitalization for a manic or mixed episode. *American Journal of Psychiatry, 155,* 646–652.

Keck, P. E., Perlis, R. H., Otto, M. W., Carpenter, D., Docherty, J. P., & Ross, R. (2004 December). Expert consensus guideline series: Treatment of bipolar disorder. *A Postgraduate Medicine Special Report,* 1–108.

Keller, M. B., Lavori, P. W., Coryell, W., Andreasen, N. C., Endicott, J., Clayton, P. J. et al. (1986). Differential outcome of pure manic, mixed/cycling, and pure depressive episodes in patients with bipolar illness. *Journal of the American Medical Association, 255,* 3138–3142.

Kessler, R. C., McGonagle, K. A., Zhao, S., Nelson, C. B., Hughes, M., Eshleman, S. et al. (1994). Lifetime and 12-month prevalence of DSM-III-r psychiatric disorders in the united states: Results from the national comorbidity survey. *Archives of General Psychiatry, 51,* 8–19.

Kim, E. Y., Miklowitz, D. J., Biuckians, A., & Mullen, K. (2007). Life stress and the course of early-onset bipolar disorder. *Journal of Affective Disorders, 99,* 37–44.

Lam, D. H., Watkins, E. R., Hayward, P., Bright, J., Wright, K., Kerr, N. et al. (2003). A randomized controlled study of cognitive therapy of relapse prevention for bipolar affective disorder: Outcome of the first year. *Archives of General Psychiatry, 60,* 145–152.

Leverich, G. S., Altshuler, L. L., Fryek Suppesk, M. A. T., Keck, P. E. Jr, McElroy, S. L., Denicoff, K. D. et al. (2003). Factors associated with suicide attempts in 648 patients with bipolar disorder in the Stanley foundation bipolar network. *Journal of Clinical Psychiatry, 64,* 506–515.

Linehan, M. M. (1993). *Cognitive-behavioral treatment of borderline personality disorder.* New York: Guilford Press.

Marangell, L. B., Bauer, M., Dennehy, E. B., Wisniewski, S., Allen, M., Miklowitz, D. et al. (2006). Prospective predictors of suicide and suicide attempts in 2000 patients with bipolar disorders followed for 2 years. *Bipolar Disorders, 8,* 566–575.

McElroy, S. L., Atshuler, L. L., Suppes, T., Keck, P. E., Frye, M. A., Denicoff, K. D. et al. (2000). Axis I psychiatric comorbidity and its relationship to historical illness variables in 288 patients with bipolar disorder. *American Journal of Psychiatry, 159,* 420–426.

McIntryre, R. S., & Konarski, J. Z. (2004). Bipolar disorder: A national health concern. *CNS Spectrums, 9*(11 Suppl 12), 6–15.

Miklowitz, D. J., George, E. L., Richards, J. A., Simoneau, T. L., & Suddath, R. L. (2003). A randomized study of family-focused psychoeducation and pharmacotherapy in the outpatient management of bipolar disorder. *Archives of General Psychiatry, 60,* 904–912.

Miklowitz, D. J., & Goldstein, M. J. (1997). *Bipolar disorder: A family-focused treatment approach.* New York: Guilford Press.

Miklowitz, D. R., Goldstein, M. J., Nuechterlein, K. H., Snyder, K. S., & Mintz, J. (1988). Family factors and the course of bipolar affective disorder. *Archives of General Psychiatry, 45,* 225–231.

Miklowitz, D. J., & Otto, M. W. (2006). New psychosocial interventions for bipolar disorder: A review of the literature and introduction of the systematic treatment enhancement program. *Journal of Cognitive Psychotherapy, 20,* 215–230.

Miklowitz, D. J., Otto, M. W., Frank, E., Reilly-Harrington, N. A., Wisniewski, S. R., Kogan, J. N. et al. (2007). Psychosocial treatments for bipolar depression: A 1-year randomized trial from the systematic treatment enhancement program. *Archives of General Psychiatry, 64,* 419–426.

Montgomery, A. (1979). A new depression scale designed to be sensitive to change. *British Journal of Psychiatry, 134,* 382–389.

Nemeroff, C. B., Evans, D. L., Gyulai, L., Sachs, G. S., Bowden, C. L., Gergel, I. P. et al. (2001). Double-blind, placebo-controlled comparison of imipramine and paroxetine in the treatment of bipolar depression. *American Journal of Psychiatry, 158,* 906–912.

Nezu, A. M., & Nezu, C. M. (1993). Identifying and selecting target problems for clinical interventions: A problem-solving model. *Psychological Assessment, 5,* 254–263.

Nierenberg, A. A., Miyahara, S., Spencer, T., Wisniewski, S. R., Otto, M. W., Pollack, M. H. et al. (2005). Clinical and diagnostic implications of lifetime ADHD comorbidity in adults with bipolar disorder: Data from the first 1000 STEP-BD participants. *Biological Psychiatry, 57,* 1467–1473.

Otto, M. W. (2000). Stories and metaphors in cognitive-behavior therapy. *Cognitive and Behavioral Practice, 7,* 166–172.

Otto, M. W., & Miklowitz, D. J. (2004). The role and impact of psychotherapy in the management of bipolar disorder. *CNS Spectrums, 9*(11 Suppl 12), 27–32.

Otto, M. W., Reilly-Harrington, N., Knauz, R. O., Henin, A., Kogan, J. N., & Sachs, G. S. (2008). *Living with bipolar disorder.* Oxford University Press.

Otto, M. W., Simon, N. S., Wisniewski, S. R., Miklowitz, D. J., Kogan, J. N., Reilly-Harrington, N. A. et al. (2006). Prospective 12-month course of bipolar disorder in outpatients with and without comorbid anxiety disorders. *British Journal of Psychiatry, 189,* 20–25.

Perlis, R. H., Miyahara, S., Marangell, L. B., Wisniewski, S. R., Ostacher, M., DelBello, M. P. et al. (2004). Long-term implications of early onset in bipolar disorder: Data from the first 1000 participants in the systematic treatment enhancement program for bipolar disorder (STEP-BD). *Biological Psychiatry, 55,* 875–881.

Perlis, R. H., Sachs, G. S., Lafer, B., Otto, M. W., Faraone, S. V., & Rosenbaum, J. F. (2002). Effect of abrupt change from standard to low serum lithium levels: A reanalysis of double-blind lithium maintenance data. *American Journal of Psychiatry, 159,* 1155–1159.

Perry, A., Tarrier, N., Morriss, R., McCarthy, E., & Limb, K. (1999). Randomised controlled trial of efficacy of teaching patients with bipolar disorder to identify early symptoms of relapse and obtain treatment. *British Medical Journal, 16,* 149–153.

Rosen, A., & Proctor, E. K. (1981). Distinctions between treatment outcomes and their implications for treatment evaluation. *Journal of Consulting and Clinical Psychology, 49,* 418–425.

Ryff, C. D., & Singer, B. (1996). Psychological well-being: Meaning, measurement, and implications. *Psychotherapy and Psychosomatics, 65,* 14–23.

Sachs, G. S., Nierenberg, A. A., Calabrese, J. R., Marangell, L. B., Wisniewski, S. R., Gyulai, L. et al. (2007). Effectiveness of adjunctive antidepressant treatment for bipolar depression. *New England Journal of Medicine, 356,* 1711–1722.

Sachs, G. S., Thase, M. E., Otto, M. W., Bauer, M., Miklowitz, D., Wisniewski, S. R. et al. (2003). Rationale, design, and methods of the systematic treatment enhancement program for bipolar disorder (STEP-BD). *Biological Psychiatry, 53,* 1028–1042.

Schneck, C. D., Miklowitz, D. J., Calabrese, J. R., Allen, M. H., Thomas, M. R., Wisniewski, S. R. et al. (2004). Phenomenology of rapid-cycling bipolar disorder: Data from the first 500 participants in the systematic treatment enhancement program. *American Journal of Psychiatry, 161,* 1902–1908.

Scott, J., Garland, A., & Moorhead, S. (2001). A pilot study of cognitive therapy in bipolar disorders. *Psychological Medicine, 31,* 459–467.

Scott, J., Paykel, E., Morriss, R., Bentall, R., Kinderman, P., Johnson, T. et al. (2006). Cognitive-behavioural therapy for severe and recurrent bipolar disorders: Randomised controlled trial. *British Journal of Psychiatry, 188,* 313–320.

Simon, N. M., Otto, M. W., Weiss, R., Bauer, M. S., Miyahara, S., Wisniewski, S. R. et al. (2004). Pharmacotherapy for bipolar disorder and comorbid conditions: Baseline data from STEP-BD. *Journal of Clinical Psychopharmacology, 24,* 512–520.

Simon, N. M., Pollack, M. H., Ostacher, M. J., Zalta, A. K., Chow, C., Fischmann, D. et al. (2007). Understanding the link between anxiety symptoms and suicidal ideation and behaviors in outpatients with bipolar disorder. *Journal of Affective Disorders, 97,* 91–99.

Weiss, R. D., Ostacher, M., Otto, M. W., Calabrese, J., Fossey, M., Wisniewski, S. R. et al. (2005). Recovery from substance use disorder in patients with bipolar disorder: Does it matter? *Journal of Clinical Psychiatry, 6,* 730–735.

Young, R. C., Biggs, J. T., Ziegler, V. E., & Meyer, D. A. (1978). A rating scale for mania: Reliability, validity, and sensitivity. *British Journal of Psychiatry, 133,* 429–435.

Zaretsky, A. E., & Segal, Z. Z. V. (1999). Cognitive therapy for bipolar depression: A pilot study. *Canadian Journal of Psychiatry, 44,* 491–494.

Zinbarg, R. E., Craske, M. G., & Barlow, D. H. (2006). *Mastery of your anxiety and worry* (2nd ed.). New York: Oxford University Press.

About the Authors

Michael W. Otto, PhD, is Professor of Psychology at Boston University and Director of the Center for Anxiety and Related Disorders. Dr. Otto specializes in the cognitive-behavioral treatment of anxiety, mood, and substance use disorders. Dr. Otto's research focuses on difficult-to-treat populations, including the application of cognitive-behavioral strategies to patients who have failed to respond to previous interventions, as well as developing novel strategies for bipolar disorder and substanceuse disorders. Regarding bipolar disorder, Dr. Otto helped direct the large-scale investigation of the efficacy of psychosocial treatments conducted as part of the federally funded Systematic Treatment Enhancement Program for Bipolar Disorder (STEP-BD). Dr. Otto has published over 250 scientific articles, chapters, and books spanning his research interests and was recently identified as a "top producer" in the clinical empirical literature. Dr. Otto is past president of the Association for Behavioral and Cognitive Therapies (formerly AABT), a fellow of the American Psychological Association, and a member of the Scientific Advisory Board for the Anxiety Disorders Association of America. Dr. Otto is richly involved in clinical training and dissemination of research findings and is a regular contributor to continuing education and continuing medical education workshops across the United States.

Noreen A. Reilly-Harrington, PhD, is a Founding Fellow of the Academy of Cognitive Therapy and is an expert in the cognitive-behavioral therapy(CBT) of mood disorders. She is a graduate of the University of Pennsylvania and Temple University and completed both her pre-doctoral internship and post-doctoral fellowship in CBT at Massachusetts General Hospital (MGH) and Harvard Medical School. Dr. Reilly-Harrington served as the Clinical and Scientific Coordinator of the Psychosocial Pathway in the NIMH STEP-BD. She has also been the Principal Investigator on two NIMH-sponsored Small Business Innovative Research projects geared at improving the design and reliability of multi-site psychiatric assessment and research. Currently, Dr. Reilly-Harrington serves as the Director of Training and Assessment for the NIMH-sponsored Bipolar Trials Network and advises the multi-site network in all aspects of protocol design, assessment selection, and training. Dr. Reilly-Harrington is also actively involved in the teaching and provision of CBT at the Massachusetts General Hospital Bipolar Clinic and Research Program and is on the faculty of Harvard Medical School.

Jane Null Kogan, PhD, is an Assistant Professor in the Department of Psychiatry at the University of Pittsburgh School of Medicine and Director of Outcomes and Research Administration at Community Care Behavioral Health, a large not-for-profit behavioral health managed care organization serving publicly and privately insured individuals across Pennsylvania. She received her PhD in Clinical Psychology from West Virginia University and completed post-doctoral training in the Department of Psychiatry at Harvard Medical School. She has been involved in numerous federally funded research grants investigating the assessment and treatment of affective disorders, including a large-scale, national effectiveness study of the treatment of bipolar disorder. In addition, she has significant experience in designing and implementing clinical research studies examining the impact of psychotherapeutic interventions for treatment of mood disorders. She is currently a coprincipal investigator on a NIMH training grant that aims to enhance the workforce of academic investigators carrying out bipolar treatment research across the United States. She is also an investigator on multiple grants examining factors that influence dissemination of evidence-based practices to community or routine care settings.

Aude Henin, PhD, is Assistant Professor of Psychology at Harvard Medical School, and Director of the Cognitive-Behavior Therapy Program in the Clinical and Research Program in Pediatric Psychopharmacology at MGH. She received her doctoral degree from Temple University and completed her pre-doctoral and post-doctoral fellowships at MGH. Dr. Henin's research focuses on the development and evaluation of psychosocial interventions for children, adolescents, and young adults with severe psychiatric and developmental disorders. She also conducts research on family studies of mood and anxiety disorders to identify risk factors for the development of these disorders in youth. Her research is funded by the NIMH and National Alliance for Research on Schizophrenia and Depression (NARSAD), and she has received several awards and honors from organizations such as the American Psychological Association, the Anxiety Disorders Association of America, and the MGH. Clinically, she specializes in CBT for children, adolescents, and young adults with mood, anxiety, and autism spectrum disorders. She also regularly lectures on the phenomenology and psychosocial treatment of childhood disorders.

Robert O. Knauz, Ph.D., is an Instructor at Harvard Medical School and a Clinical Assistant at MGH in Boston. He is also the Clinical Coordinator at the Behavioral Medicine Service at MGH and a consultant at Concordant Rater Systems, devoted to research training and the accurate use of assessments to measure mood and anxiety disorders. He received his PhD. in Clinical Psychology at the University of Massachusetts, Amherst, and completed his post-doctoral training in the Department of Psychiatry at Harvard Medical School. He has an extensive clinical background in Bipolar Disorder and in Behavioral Medicine. He was part of the STEP-BD and examined the efficacy of several psychological treatments for Bipolar Disorder. Dr. Knauz was also the coprincipal investigator on 2 NIMH and The Health Resources and Services Administration (HRSA) funded grants examining the effectiveness of a novel treatment to reduce secondary rates of HIV infection. Dr. Knauz has trained physicians, psychiatrists, psychologists and other clinicians both nationally and internationally on the diagnosis of Bipolar Disorder and more accurate ways of assessing the symptoms of this disease.

Gary S. Sachs, MD, is Associate Professor of Psychiatry at Harvard Medical School and director of the Bipolar Clinic and Research Program at MGH. Dr. Sachs' research focuses on bipolar disorder, particularly clinical trial methodology, effectiveness studies, and development of collaborative chronic disease management models. His current research projects include studies of novel treatments for bipolar depression and interventions for ineffective complex cases as well as chronic care models. He served as Principal investigator of the STEP-BD. Dr. Sachs is a Distinguished Fellow of the American Psychiatric Association. He is chair of the Scientific Advisory Board of the National Alliance on Mental Illness and serves on the Scientific Advisory Board of the Depression and Bipolar Support Alliance. Dr. Sachs is coeditor-in-chief of *Clinical Approaches to Bipolar Disorder* and is actively involved in teaching trainees and postgraduate education. He has authored over 150 articles, abstracts, books, reviews, and book chapters. Dr. Sachs now leads the Collaborative Care Initiative at MGH.

Printed in Great Britain
by Amazon.co.uk, Ltd.,
Marston Gate.